BOVINE SCIENCE - A KEY TO SUSTAINABLE DEVELOPMENT

Edited by **Sadashiv S. O.**
and **Sharangouda J. Patil**

Bovine Science - A Key to Sustainable Development
http://dx.doi.org/10.5772/intechopen.73743
Edited by Sadashiv S. O. and Sharangouda J. Patil

Contributors

Borisz Egri, Antonio Pérez, Karla Quintal, Teresa Espinosa, Muhammad Khalid Bashir, Bahar-E Mustafa, Shahid Ur-Rehman, Muhammad Ashraf, Muhammad Adnan Ashraf, Nazir Ahmad, Muhammad Kamran Khan, Muhammad Imran, Muhammad Nadeem Suleman, Sufyan Afzal, Henny Nuraini, Edit Lesa Aditia, Bram Brahmantiyo, Sadashiv S. O.

Notice

Statements and opinions expressed in the chapters are these of the individual contributors and not necessarily those of the editors or publisher. No responsibility is accepted for the accuracy of information contained in the published chapters. The publisher assumes no responsibility for any damage or injury to persons or property arising out of the use of any materials, instructions, methods or ideas contained in the book.

First published in London, United Kingdom, 2019 by IntechOpen
IntechOpen is the global imprint of INTECHOPEN LIMITED, registered in England and Wales, registration number: 11086078, The Shard, 25th floor, 32 London Bridge Street
London, SE19SG – United Kingdom
Printed in Croatia

British Library Cataloguing-in-Publication Data
A catalogue record for this book is available from the British Library

Additional hard copies can be obtained from orders@intechopen.com

Bovine Science - A Key to Sustainable Development, Edited by Sadashiv S. O. and Sharangouda J. Patil
p. cm.
Print ISBN 978-1-78985-605-7
Online ISBN 978-1-78985-606-4

We are IntechOpen,
the world's leading publisher of
Open Access books
Built by scientists, for scientists

4,000+
Open access books available

116,000+
International authors and editors

120M+
Downloads

151
Countries delivered to

Our authors are among the

Top 1%
most cited scientists

12.2%
Contributors from top 500 universities

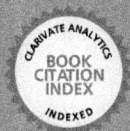

Interested in publishing with us?
Contact book.department@intechopen.com

Numbers displayed above are based on latest data collected.
For more information visit www.intechopen.com

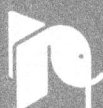

Meet the editors

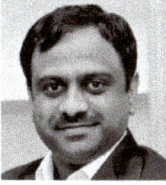

Dr. Sadashiv S. O. is currently working as an Assistant Professor in the Department of Life Sciences, Garden City University, Bengaluru, Karnataka, India. He has obtained his Masters and Ph D. in Microbiology from Karnatak University, Dharwad. He has published 19 research articles in peer-reviewed national and international journals, 2 books, 5 book chapters and has edited 3 books. He has successfully guided various projects for Masters and Ph.D. students. He has secured two Young Scientists Award, one Gold Medal award and an Appreciation Award from the Zoological Society of India, for contribution in the field of microbiology. He has also worked in various academic responsibilities such as Editor in Chief, Advisory Editorial Member for various journals, BOS, BOE and a Coordinator for UG/PG examinations. His main areas of research are molecular biology, animal biotechnology and medical microbiology.

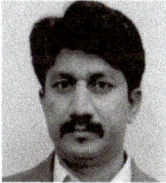

Dr. Sharangouda J. Patil was born and brought up in a farming community. Due to his strong will and aspiration for teaching and research, he overcame several limitations to develop himself as an eminent researcher and teacher. He has successfully guided various projects for Masters and Ph.D. students. Currently he is working as an Associate Professor at the School of Science, Garden City University, Bangalore. During his academic career, he has published more than 55 research articles, 4 book chapters, 5 technical bulletins and several other technical articles in national and international journals. He has participated in and presented research papers in more than 70 conferences and has been awarded many best paper awards. Dr. Patil is also working as an Editor in Chief, Editorial Board Member, Advisory Editorial Member and a Reviewer to more than 35 journals. His efforts as a teacher and researcher have proved him a man of diverse skills, who aspires to set up an academic culture and educational program conducive to student learning and progress.

Contents

Preface

Since the beginning of civilization, humans and animals developed very strong associations to their mutual benefits. The lives of humans and animals have been connected in all aspects. Early humans learned to raise animals for food and this continues today. Ruminant livestock are the most domesticated animals that includes bovines, ovines and caprines. Livestock, particularly bovines, are important contributors to total food production in the world. Moreover, their contribution increases at a higher rate than that of cereals. These animals play very important economic and socio-cultural roles for the welfare of rural households. They help in employment, soil fertility, livelihoods, transport, agricultural traction, agricultural diversification, food supply, source of income and also in sustainable agricultural production. These animals play an important role in food supply for rural and urban areas and contribute to family nutrition. Products such as milk, eggs, and meat are used as a source of food, with other livestock products used for domestic consumption.

The social expectations in Science and Technology are increasing because of rapid advances. Prevention and control of infectious diseases in bovines have been among the top-most public health objectives in the last decades. However, controlling diseases due to pathogens that move between animals and humans remains challenging. Such pathogens have been responsible for the majority of new human and bovine disease threats as was proved with a number of recent international epidemic incidences. Identifying and addressing emergent cross-species infections will require a newer approach, in which resources from public veterinary, environmental and human health functions as a part of an integrative system.

The current technological boom has put forth a variety of research techniques, methods and protocols being used in bovine science. There is now a great deal of interaction between the chemical, physical and biological sciences. Nutritional management is required in bovines, as it is an important criterion to match the current increasing need of the population. Meeting with such issues, dietary requirements maximize production and hence profit potential and minimizes soil, water, diseases and atmospheric impacts. The biologist today depends on recent advances of bovine science in aspects of physiology, biochemistry, microbiology, biotechnology, genetics, pharmacology, toxicology and environmental biology of these animals. Several technologies have been developed over the years to address the challenges of bovine science. This book is aimed at young researchers, academicians and industry people.

In this book, experts from different continents present some of the important aspects of bovine science such as louse infestations of ruminants, cytogenetics of bovines, factors of competitiveness for the bovine livestock, bovine feed manipulation, enhancement of conjugated linoleic acid and its bioavailability, emergence of antimicrobial resistance, prevention strategies and meat quality. The aim of this book to give an understanding of the present scenario, advances, and challenges in bovine science.

This book is dedicated to all academicians and researchers.

Dr. Sadashiv S. O. and Dr. Sharangouda J. Patil
School of Sciences
Department of Life Sciences
Garden City University
Bengaluru, Karnataka, India

Chapter 1

Introductory Chapter: Bovine Science - A Key to Sustainable Development

Sadashiv S.O. and Sharangouda J. Patil

Additional information is available at the end of the chapter

http://dx.doi.org/10.5772/intechopen.83723

1. Introduction

1.1. Livestock

Livestock animals play vital role in socio-economic, cultural and these animals serve as a function for rural households. Livestock helps in food supply, family nutrition, quality savings, family financial gain, increase in soil productivity, livelihoods, transport, agricultural diversification and production, family and community employment, ritual functions, and social station. As per the Food and Agriculture Organization (FAO), two widely used classifications are supported the forms of output created or inside the uses [1].

Among output uses, maintenance and consumption by the farm holder's house, direct offer of inputs, financial gain through sales of the live animals or their output, savings investment and social functions like paying bride wealth, or in other way providing animals for communal feasts or sacrifices will be distinguished. Another classification divides animal functions in the economic role like supply of financial gain and mean of savings accumulation, direct feed use for family subsistence, additional benefits like fertilizer and animal draught, and capability to accommodate a collection of social rules and obligations. Livestock has a crucial contribution to the food chain of rural and urban areas and contributes to family nutrition. As a social unit, financial gain will increase and consumption of product will increase, mainly from animal origin, permitting the substitution of vegetal diet by animal supermolecule. Apart from milk, eggs, and meat used in food, skins, hides, and horns are also used for domestic purposes.

Livestock production is closely reticulated with crop production. The employment of livestock and its by-product manure are widely used in crop production. It may be a supply of energy, providing draught animal power, and manure improves soil structure and fertility and also increases water retention. Each use is environmentally friendly and yields more energy and nutrient support. Its production is a very important mean of exchange between rural households and, when sold, contributes to spice up and strengthen the rural markets. Rural markets are very important areas within the operation mode of rural communities and play a big contribution for rural families in the upgradation of wealth. Livestock may feature as savings and may be regenerated into money whenever the family desires it; also it may act as a security, influencing access to informal credits and loans and being conjointly a supply of collateral for loans. In many rural regions, wherever monetary markets are absent or nonexistent, livestock's or herds are a supply of plus accumulation and live of prosperity. Livestock or assets may be mobilized at any time, satisfying planned expenditures, for example, kids' fees and bride wealth, or many unplanned expenses like the unhealthiness and death of members of the family. These animals may well be seen as a "bank account," and they are conjointly a very important supply of family savings that may be employed in years of low crop production, reducing financial insecurity and social unit vulnerability, being a very important supply of risk reduction and security increase.

Animal health greatly affects the farm animal functions, not solely by direct effects on animal productivity but also by indirect effects, specifically regarding human health, costs associated to disease management, and international movement restrictions of animals on animal merchandise and animal welfare [2]. The existence of an excellent variety of parasitary, infectious, or metabolic diseases that have an effect on fertility cannot be underestimated. Besides the positive effects of stock to human welfare, stock production and consumption may be associated with some risks, specifically the transmission of vital diseases that are transmitted from animals to humans (zoonosis). The absence of rigorous animal health management programs represents a high risk to the human health. Furthermore, the rigorous management and restrictions to animal movement and to exportation of animal merchandise, related to the existence of disease, makes the existence of national animal health programs indispensable so as to permit international trade.

2. Bovine mastitis

Bovine mastitis in farm cows may be a significant issue because it is an economically devastating sickness inflicting large economic losses within the farm trade and is the worldwide costliest production unwellness in dairy farm herds. It stands second to foot and mouth disease as the most difficult disease in high-yielding dairy farm animals in Asian countries; however, as per reports of the prevalence of mastitis in dairy farm animals, it stands on initial position and had been reported quite in a high rate in crossbred dairy farms. Field surveys of major placental mammal diseases have indicated that inflammation is one of the foremost major diseases of farm animals [3].

Mastitis is the outcome of interaction of assorted factors related to the host, pathogen(s), and therefore the atmosphere. Infectious agents, particularly varied species of bacterium, are the foremost vital etiologic agents of inflammation. The association of some host, management, and housing determinants with inflammation is well-established and was the subject of investigation. Bovine inflammation is caused by the entry of bacterium within the mammary gland resulting in inflammation. This illness, characterized by a rise in the cells, particularly leukocytes, within the milk and by pathological changes within the mammary gland tissue, causes large economic losses and additionally holds the danger for the transmission of animal diseases like TB, brucellosis, and zoonotic disease. Bovine mastitis is generally classified into clinical and subclinical mastitis. Clinical mastitis is characterized by local (e.g., swelling of the udder, heat, and pain) or systemic (e.g., fever, anorexia, depression) symptoms with milk abnormalities (e.g., milk clots, flakes, watery secretions, blood). Subclinical redness is that the most serious kind because the infected animal shows no obvious symptoms and secrets apparently traditional milk for an extended time, therefore it is a crucial feature of the medical specialty of bovine inflammation.

The consumption of dairy farm product has additionally magnified at similar levels with a great increase in recent years, primarily because of a bigger income base for people. Improving udder health and decreasing the incidence of udder infection and inflammation in dairy farm herds can end in augmented milk production. Even though advanced technology is created, mastitis continues to be a significant economic issue for dairy farm producers. Thus, researchers and dairy farm advisors still refine the National Mastitis Council (NMC) and regularly they counsel farm producers on mastitis management program.

Increase in the prevalence of mastitis might be due to the absence of udder washing and milking of cows with common milkers which have cuts and chaps on their hands and using of common udder cloths, which could be vectors of spread especially for contagious mastitis. In the preparation for milking, teats and udder should be properly washed with suitable sanitizing agent and completely dried, even before and after milking to control mastitis effectively. In order to reduce the high prevalence of bovine mastitis, improved milking hygiene, hindrance of skin lesions, culling of chronic mastitis carriers, and treating of clinically infected herds must be practiced. Improper hygiene and poor farm management practices contributed to the presence of many pathogenic bacteria in milk. Improving the hygienic conditions of the milking environment and utensils may reduce the prevalence of many pathogens in milk, and also implementation of a systematic application of an in vitro antibiotic susceptibility test, earlier to the use of antibiotics in both treatment and prevention of bovine mastitis, is reommended [4].

3. Feed and fodder management

The previous report of five year plan of the animal husbandry, agriculture, horticulture and forestry departments, with slight intersectoral conversation between these departments in around the world for the fodder production and management. Livestock farming is one of the major occupations of farmers along with or without agriculture and entrepreneurs to produce various products for the tremendous input to the country's gross domestic product (GDP). Livestock farming is one of the important livestock activities worldwide to produce and provide milk, meat, manure, leather, wool, energy for agriculture, basic transportation, and many useful food sources and income-generating works for millions of households throughout the world [5].

The number of livestock from the past few years has increased in all the conditions, in the form of two levels, i.e., (i) maximum number of farmers practicing extensive stall feeding in different breeds of hybrid cattle and (ii) similarly also increased grazing of local variety livestock population to depend their survival on the natural sources. Increasing livestock population without information is against to the animal husbandry policies, without attention of their feed and fodder sources, production of feed and fodder should be in farms by scientific management, otherwise, it is stress on the livestock and if sources are limited, poor fodder production technologies and storage methods in the developed country to depleting productivity sources of the farming area.

The annual estimated growth and income depends on urbanization, globalization, and civilization of the countries, demand for the livestock resources also increased subsequently, and further research is required for future advancements in production of animal products to meet the demand of global population. In 2050, the global demand for dairy and meat products are expected to increase by 74 % and 58 %, respectively, by the choice of developing countries. The cattle global population in 2000 was 1.5 billion and many model projects by the government are helping to the increase by 2050 at around 2.7 and 2.6 billion, respectively. For this, animal feed ingredient requirement is estimated to increase annually by 553 million tonnes; it was also reported by the FAO in 2009 that 50% of the demand were met in that year [6]. To meet the future demands of global population, the production of milk and meat strategies need to be depends on animal health, food & nutrition and scientific management by using available feed and fodder resources, also they are monitored all the time for serve the livestock sufficient and significantly [7].

Strategies are also required to improve feed quality, fodder resources, and sustainability in management of livestock production. It is necessary to adopt newer technology of fodder production to utilize it efficiently and effectively without wasting the available natural resources for improvement in productivity of the future food security of the country. Management and practices came through traditional approach, they are modified into modern technologies for high yield variety of green fodder production, different strategies to enhance fodder production/unit land area and using locally available resources. To livestock farmers, encourage and promote high yield varieties for fodder production in integrated farming systems along with agriculture and horticulture practices. Livestock farmers adopt the waste and barren land resources for cultivation of fodders, it will shows the conservation strategies of the biodiversity for the establishment of diverse agro-forest ecosystem. Available resources of agriculture like crop residues and by products of the agriculture and horticulture utilize it as a feeds and fodders. Introduce the newer technologies of research institutes/industries in the field level to manage systematically and to enhance the fodder production. Governments organization like FAO, ICRISAT, ILRI, IFAD, ICAR, CABI, IRRI, IRRD working on feed and fodder resources for scale up as per the requirement and modification in the fodder production processes, come out with best viable and economic products. There is a proper attention in the area of fodder production by introducing improved variety of high-yielding fodders (varieties of grasses and leguminous), perennial fodder trees and shrubs & herbs to make sure there is sufficiently available food to feed for livestock across the year. In this context, the production of feed and fodder depends on quality seeds sapling material and scientific information and there availability to the farmers.

The concept of conservation of feed and fodder for sustainable development seems to be a newer approach for most of the farmers. Application of new technologies to make the feed and fodder to store in limited spaces and equipped with low cost conservation strategies like box baling, silage making to use it in scarcity time for livestock [8]. For dry fodder, conserve as feed block preparation using different dry fodders with enriched nutrients or balanced ration, urea treatment of straws, degradation by enzymatic action, etc.

The recently investigated newer technique called "hydroponics" means growing fodder plant material using the required environment with nutrients, desired temperature, and humidity in water without soil. Hydroponics is an easier and faster technology to produce green fodder to maintain livestock production all the time. Maize is the potential seed source for hydroponics, and even cowpea, chickpea, grams, hemps, and any millet seeds can be grown in very limited amount of time with maximum production. By the literature, hydroponics yield differs with the type of crop, for example, ragi and bajra ranging from 300%, maize, cowpea, and grams were 600%, and sun hemp was 800%. Based on nutritional parameters, a leguminous crop was used for production and it is encouraging as rich fodder crop with high crude content of protein than the cereal and millet crops. Hydroponic fodder is a highly enriched nutritional feed to livestock and is found to be highly palatable with 100% utilization with proper management [9].

These management plans will useful for bovines and it is depends on utilization of the available feed and fodder resources timely to get quality products and supply for the use of human population.

Author details

Sadashiv S.O.* and Sharangouda J. Patil

*Address all correspondence to: sadashivso@gmail.com

School of Sciences, Department of Life Sciences, Garden City University, Bengaluru, Karnataka, India

References

[1] Bettencourt EMV, Tilman M, Narciso V, da Silva Carvalho ML, de Sousa Henriques PD. The livestock roles in the wellbeing of rural communities of Timor-Leste. Revista de Economia e Sociologia Rural. 2015;**53**(1):S063-S080

[2] Otte MJ, Chilonda P. Animal Health Economics: An Introduction. Rome, Italy: Livestock Information, Sector Analysis and Policy Branch, Animal Production and Health Division, FAO; 2000

[3] Sadashiv SO, Kaliwal BB. Resistance in bacteria. In: Insecticides Resistance. Rijeka, Crotia: InTech; 2016. pp. 295-312. DOI: 10.5772/61479. 978-953-51-2258-6

[4] Sadashiv SO, Kaliwal BB. Screening and antibiotic resistance of *Escherichia coli* isolated from bovine mastitis in the region of North Karnataka, India. Indo American Journal of Pharmaceutical Research. 2015;5(4):1309-1316

[5] Anon. Issues for the Approach to the 12th Plan. India: Planning Commission of India; 2011

[6] FAO. The State of Food and Agriculture. Rome, Italy: Livestock in the Balance; 2009

[7] FAO. In: Garg MR, editor. Balanced Feeding for Improving Livestock Productivity — Increase in Milk Production and Nutrient Use Efficiency and Decrease in Methane Emission. Vol. 173. Rome, Italy: FAO Animal Production and Health; 2012

[8] Lukuyu B, Franzel S, Ongadi PM, Duncan AJ. Livestock feed resources: Current production and management practices in central and northern rift valley provinces of Kenya. Livestock Research for Rural Development. 2011;23(5):112

[9] Jemimah ER, Gnanaraj PT, Muthuramalingam T, Devi T. Hydroponic Green Fodder Production — TANUVAS Experience. Tamilnadu, India: National Agricultural Development Programme (NADP); 2015. pp. 1-77

Chapter 2

Factors of Competitiveness for the Bovine Livestock in Yucatan, Mexico

Antonio Emmanuel Perez Brito,
Teresa de Jesus Espinosa Atoche and
Karla Patricia Quintal Gordillo

Additional information is available at the end of the chapter

http://dx.doi.org/10.5772/intechopen.79305

Abstract

This chapter's objective is to show that finance, marketing and innovation could be considered as factors of competitiveness. Owners of 30 cattle ranches were included in the state surveys, with each ranch having at least 1000 head of cattle. The study was quantitative and used a multiple linear regression model. The results were that the use of financial information, the profitability and funding are components of finance factor. The product and the process innovation are components of innovation factor and the market positioning, the knowledge of the competition and customer satisfaction are components of marketing factor, being the profitability, the market positioning, the customer satisfaction, the product and the process innovation, relatively more important.

Keywords: bovine livestock, competitiveness, finance, innovation, marketing, Mexico

1. Introduction

Meat is an important element in human nutrition and, in the world dietary context, the level of consumption is an indicator of the life of the population [1].

In Ref. [2], livestock represents 40% of the global value of agricultural production and the basis of livelihoods and food security of almost one billion people. The livestock sector, driven by the increase in income and support of technological and structural changes, is the fastest-growing in the agricultural economy. The progress and transformation of the sector offer opportunities for agricultural development, but the rapid pace of change could marginalize small farmers; on the other hand, it must address systemic risks to the environment and human health with a view to ensuring sustainability.

In Ref. [3], mentioned that livestock activity in Mexico is carried out throughout the country; he affirmed that 56% of the national territory is dedicated to livestock, approximately 110 million hectares.

Livestock breeding takes place in four large areas: the arid and semi-arid, the humid tropics, the temperate and subhumid tropics [4].

In Ref. [5], it was indicated that in the state of Yucatan, the agricultural and fishing sector represent 6.7% of the total Gross Domestic Product in the state.

In Ref. [4], it was mentioned that the livestock is composed of the following products: cattle, sheep, horses, pigs, poultry, turkeys and bees.

Cattle ranching in the state of Yucatan constitutes a relevant economic activity because it occupies about 30% of Yucatan territory. The authors indicate that the eastern zone of the state of Yucatan has the largest concentration of cattle. The municipalities located in the eastern region are Sucilá, Espita, San Felipe, Panabá, Tizimín, Buctzotz, Cenotillo and Valladolid, with Tizimín constituting 90% of cattle production [6].

The agricultural sector in Yucatan faces several challenges: disorganization of beef producers in the region; problems in the integration of the various links in the production-consumption chain [7]; unemployment resulting from limited job opportunities, resulting in labor migration to other regions [8]; lack of effective marketing strategies to ensure higher sales, market diversification, and the use of intermediaries in marketing [9]; lack of technology, knowledge, and limited financial resources to generate innovation in production units, value-generation for all activities; and finally, market competitiveness [10].

The eastern zone has an area of 413,237 ha. It occupies 11% of Yucatan territory; in some parts, there is still vegetation rich in precious woods. It is also noted that the zone has fertile land capable of producing many kinds of tropical fruit [5].

In Ref. [5], the economically active population numbers 43,256 people, of whom 21,280 are reported as employed.

The census also reports that the income per person of the population is low. Of the total employed population, 14,111 people receive a salary between one and two minimum wages and only 3210 people receive more than five minimum wages. The latter figure corresponds to people working in the capital city of Mérida and in some other locations in the state of Quintana Roo. For this reason, the eastern region of the state of Yucatan is considered to be in extreme poverty.

In Ref. [5], the income of the employed population by sector is integrated as follows: 8205 people obtain income from the primary sector, 4114 from the secondary sector, and 8961 from the tertiary sector, which is saturated and provides less and less income to those who engage in the above activities.

An important business market to consider taking advantage of the proximity to it is the state of Quintana Roo. In Ref. [11], reports that in order to meet the rapidly increasing demand, Quintana Roo needs to obtain agricultural and livestock products from outside its borders to feed its growing tourism industry and atypical demography.

The general objective of this research is to generate a competitiveness index based on three factors: finance, innovation and marketing.

2. Literature review, methodology and results

2.1. Literature review

2.1.1. Competitiveness

In [12], it was noted that technological change could affect competition in virtually any activity. The impact of technology on competitiveness occurs because it affects differentiation or cost, the two fundamental generic strategies.

The competitiveness of a company is represented by the payment of higher wages, better jobs and greater safety for workers in the plant and the surroundings [13].

In [14], it was pointed out that it is also necessary to consider a very important factor that can cause the customer to value the product of the company more: having products to complement the main products of the company. These complementers can also become competitive products over time.

In [15], it was indicated that organizations would be competitive only to the extent that the products and services they offer have the attributes that correspond to the key purchasing criteria of a substantial number of customers.

In [16], it was remarked that companies that have managed to survive have resorted to competitiveness as a fundamental element. Competitiveness depends more and more on the way in which economic agents organize themselves into networks of companies that cooperate and compete with each other. Agricultural activity is not exempt from being immersed in today's globalization.

According to Blunck [17], competitiveness is the ability to provide products and services in a more efficient and effective way than competitors. In the commercial sector, this entails sustained success in international markets without protection or subsidies. Competitiveness at the industry level is the best indicator of the economic health of nations that compete at the enterprise level.

In [18], it was concluded in a study on competitiveness in the coffee industry in Veracruz that the factors that lead to greater incidence of it are as follows:

1. innovation,

2. marketing,

3. finances

In [19], it was established that the only way to be competitive is through maintaining advantages in innovation in the long term, and the only way to achieve this is by investing in new differentiated capacities.

According to Malhotra and Manyika [20], for companies to be competitive, it is necessary that governments at the federal, state and local levels effectively address the broad barriers that hinder productivity growth and support innovation in companies.

2.1.2. Innovation as a factor of competitiveness

According to Porter [21], companies achieve competitiveness through acts of innovation, which include both new technologies and new ways of doing things (innovation of products and processes).

Several innovations create competitive advantages by perceiving a completely new market opportunity or by serving a market segment that others have ignored. Competitive advantages are generated when competitors are slow to respond to innovations.

In international markets, the author points out that innovations that generate competitive advantage must anticipate both domestic and external needs.

Information plays an important role in the process of innovation and improvement. Sometimes this information comes from simple investments in research and development or market research.

With few exceptions, innovation is the result of an unusual effort. The company that successfully implements a new or better way to compete pursues its approach with a single-minded determination, often in the face of harsh criticism and difficult obstacles. Indeed, to be successful, innovation usually requires pressure, necessity, and sometimes adversity; the fear of losing often provides more impetus than the hope of winning.

Once the company reaches the competitive advantage through innovation, it can only sustain it with persistent, continuous improvement.

Competitors will eventually and inevitably surpass any company that stops the processes of improvement and innovation. Sometimes the advantage of being the first, for example in customer relationships, economies of scale in existing technologies or loyalty of distribution channels, is not enough to allow a stagnant company to retain its entrenched position for years or even for decades; sooner or later, more dynamic rivals will find a way to innovate around those advantages or create a better or more economical way of doing things.

Ultimately, the same author establishes that in order to sustain a competitive advantage over time, it is necessary to stay up to date.

According to Schroeder [22], innovation should be considered as a boost to the market, making what can be sold; impulse to technology, selling what can be done; and inter-functional, seeking cooperation between the different areas involved. The steps to follow in an innovation process are focused on the generation of the idea, product selection, preliminary design of the proto-type, prototype construction, testing and definitive design of the product, which will stimulate competitiveness in organizations, that is, in a continuous research and development to innovate.

In [23], the global competitiveness index assumes that, in the first stage of development, the economy of a country is driven by a series of factors such as unskilled labor and, above all, natural resources. This is when the four elements (institutions, labor, macroeconomic envi-ronment and infrastructure) play an important role in what has been called factor-driven economies.

2.1.3. Marketing as a factor of competitiveness

The competitive behavior of marketing is the rivalry between companies expressed in market strategies; that is, when a firm reacts to the marketing actions of a competitor in a certain way. There are three ways to react or competitive behavior: revengeful, cooperative and base or opportunistic. The first type of behavior is an aggressive response to an attack; the second consists of actions of the same type and in the same direction, but they are not perceived as aggressive by the competitor. The third behavior occurs when a company reduces its market-ing effort and competitors take advantage of that decision [24].

According to Galán and Vecino [25], there is a certain consensus among researchers to point out that the competitiveness of the company is determined by three types of factors or sources: those related to the country where the company is located (country effect or territory effect), derivatives of the sector to which it belongs (sector effect or industry effect) and those that have their origin in the company itself (company effect).

According to Stanton et al. [26], market positioning is the proportion of total sales of a product during a certain period in a specific market captured by a company. Similarly, it can also be considered as the potential part of the market that a company plans to achieve on the sales volume that all companies that sell a product during a certain period can expect to sell under ideal conditions.

In [27], it was pointed out that marketing implies knowledge of the competition and creates pricing policies and customer satisfaction services.

Accordingly, Fischer and Espejo [28] pointed out that the benefits that marketing brings to a company can be many and diverse: it contributes directly to sales, innovates products and services, satisfies the changing needs of the consumer, contributes to raise the profits of the company and generates great benefits in organizations.

2.1.4. Finance as a factor of competitiveness

The financial resources serve to maintain the solvency of the company in supplying necessary cash flows to satisfy the obligations and acquire the circulating assets necessary to achieve the objectives of the company and improve the competitiveness. In order to have financial resources, it is necessary to measure profitability and financing in companies [29].

The use of financial information is indispensable in the implementation and development of strategies in organizations. This same author establishes that financial institutions are willing to lend funds for projects that are profitable and that guarantee the recovery of said funds [30].

In [31], it was pointed out that the maintenance of good financial standards through proper financial management is one of the main factors highlighted as necessary to achieve competitive success. In this sense, it is necessary to carry out short-term planning with caution, implement and control information systems, pay special attention to credit institutions, establish annual budgets, analyze the economic-financial situation and try to measure possible, use own sources of financing. To develop the aforementioned [32], comment that the level of education to be a reflection of knowledge and skills possessed, is positively related to the ability of the manager to make strategic choices according to the demands of the environment, with its propensity to generate and implement creative solutions to the problems of the entity and even with the highest level of productivity [33].

Companies have many objectives, but according to Sallenave [34], they can be reduced to three: profitability, growth and survival. Until the 1970s, emphasis was placed on profitability; in the 1970s and 1980s, growth was sought, and today survival is sought. The latter presupposes the previous two. Without profitability and growth, there is no survival.

This same author points out that there are three fundamental characteristics of profitability (ROS), profitability over assets (ROA) and financial profitability (ROE).

According to David [30], the companies that apply the most profitable and more successful management concepts than those that do not, register more sales and reach higher levels of productivity and competitiveness. The companies that do not arrive at anything tend to carry out myopic activities and do not show well the forecasts of the future activities.

2.2. Methodology

In the present investigation, a type of quantitative research was applied because a correlation was applied, for which a Pearson statistical analysis was carried out. This study is based on the temporal dimension of the cross section. It is not experimental, because it seeks to determine the processes that lead cattle producers in the state of Yucatan to improve and generate value, thereby increasing competitiveness. The study was carried out in 2014.

For the determination of the competitiveness index, the research work used information obtained by the large ranching operations (at least 1000 head of cattle) in the state of Yucatan in 2014. A survey was applied specifically to obtained needed information for this investigation.

In Ref. [35], the study population was made up of 30 large ranches in the state of Yucatan. In this case, all the observation units that make up the target population could be accessed.

The validity and reliability of the recruitment instrument was reviewed mainly through the exhaustive review of the literature, the content validity, the validity of construction, through the application of the factorial analysis and the reliability analysis of the instrument by the Cronbach alpha coefficient.

2.2.1. Validity

Content: the validity of content has been achieved by reviewing the literature on the subject that has shaped the theoretical framework of the research, as well as the review and adaptation of the recruitment instrument, after reviewing it by the experts. The uptake instrument was previously applied in a similar study in the state of Sonora [36].

Construction: the validity of the construction of the collection instrument was determined through the application of factor analysis in [37], on the content variables related to the marketing, innovation and finance sections. The results obtained for each section are presented below (see **Table 1**).

According to the results, the KMO sample adequacy coefficient is considered acceptable for all cases higher than 0.7, a value that several authors [38], consider adequate for the application of factor analysis. On the other hand, the value of the Bartlett test is based on the hypothesis of an inadequate relationship between the variables for the application of the analysis, so this relationship is considered adequate, and the application of the factor analysis is relevant. On the other hand, in all three cases, the first component explains a percentage close to 70% or greater, so that the variables can be considered to be in a group around the corresponding construct (marketing, innovation and finance). The results obtained by applying the IBM SPPP Statistics 21 statistical package.

2.2.2. Reliability measurement

Reliability can be measured by using a measuring instrument or more times with the same group of people or by applying two or more measuring instruments to the same group at different times. The split halves method requires only one application of the measurement and comparison of the parts that must be highly correlated. The Cronbach alpha coefficient requires only one measurement administration for the whole population without the need to divide it.

The method used for the characteristics of the research is the Cronbach coefficient.

$$\alpha = \frac{NP}{(1+P(N-1))} \tag{1}$$

where α=Cronbach's alpha reliability coefficient; N = number of items; P = average of the correlations between items.

Considering that the content reagents are presented on a Likert scale, to establish the reliability of the capturing instrument, Cronbach's alpha coefficient was applied for each of the

Section	KMO coefficient	P value of the Bartlett test	Explained percentage of variance
Marketing	0.833	0.000	74.5
Innovation	0.728	0.000	80.3
Finance	0.825	0.000	68.9

Source: Own elaboration based on research data.

Table 1. Validation results of the instrument's construct.

Section	Cronbach's alpha coefficient
Marketing	0.974
Innovation	0.984
Finance	0.960
General	0.989

Source: Own elaboration based on research data.

Table 2. Reliability analysis.

sections (marketing, innovation and finance) and for the complete instrument. The results are presented in **Table 2**.

According to the results, for any of the sections, the value of the Cronbach alpha coefficient is greater than 0.95, so that once the reliability was tested per section, the value of the coefficient for the complete instrument was obtained. This turned out to be 0.983, a value which supports the affirmation that the capture instrument is reliable. The results were obtained by applying the IBM SPPP Statistics 21 statistical package.

2.3. Results

Prior to the construction of the competitiveness indicator, the possible existence of atypical data was analyzed through the construction of a box diagram [39], for the sums of the reagent ratings associated with the sections corresponding to marketing, innovation, and finance. As a result, the nonexistence of extreme values was confirmed.

Since the statistical results of the study correspond to a population, the run test [40] was applied to determine if the sums per section could be considered as random. According to the p values obtained for this test (0.593, 0.193 and 0.193) for a significance level of 0.05, the randomness hypothesis cannot be rejected, so it is confirmed that the results can be considered random. Similar results were obtained for the indices that were subsequently constructed using the threshold method (see **Tables 3** and **4**).

	Sum of Section 2	Sum of Section 3	Sum of Section 4
Median	51	181	92
Cases < median	14	15	15
Cases ≥median	16	15	15
Total cases	30	30	30
Number of streaks	14	12	12
Z value	−.535	−1.301	−1.301
P values	.593	.193	.193

Source: Own elaboration based on research data.

Table 3. Streak test by section.

	Marketing indicator	Innovation indicator	Finance indicator	Competitiveness indicator
Median	60.0	52.0	49.0	53.7
Cases < median	14	15	15	15
Cases ≥median	16	15	15	15
Total cases	30	30	30	30
Number of streaks	18	18	18	18
Z value	.585	.557	.557	.557
P value	.559	.577	.577	.577

Source: Own elaboration based on research data.

Table 4. Streak test by factor.

Likewise, the Kolmogorov–Smirnov goodness-of-fit test was applied to establish whether the results of the indicators could be considered to have a normal distribution. According to the p-values obtained for this test (0.06, 0.180, 0.595 and 0.114), for a level of significance of 0.05, the normality hypothesis cannot be rejected, so it is confirmed that the values of the indicators have this distribution (see **Table 5**).

To establish the competitiveness index of the observation units under study, the Marketing, Innovation and Finance indices were previously obtained, considering that the response to the reagents is presented on an additive Likert scale, using the threshold method [41], according to which the value of the index in scale from 0 to 100 for the ith observation is obtained by the expression:

$$Ind_i = \left(\frac{x_i - x_{min}}{x_{máx} - x_{mín}} \right) \times 100 \qquad (2)$$

		Marketing indicator	Innovation indicator	Finance indicator	Competitiveness indicator
N		30	30	30	30
Descriptive measures	Mean	49.444	38.026	37.949	41.999
	Standard deviation	26.3099	25.8404	21.9028	24.2776
More extreme differences	Absolute	.241	.200	.140	.218
	Positive	.140	.150	.140	.161
	Negative	−.241	−.200	−.130	−.218
Z value		1.323	1.097	.769	1.196
P values		.060	.180	.595	.114

Source: Own elaboration based on research data.

Table 5. Kolmogorov-Smirnov test for a simple.

where Ind_i It is the value of the Indicator (marketing, innovation, finance) for the ith observation unit; x_i It is the sum of the rating awarded for the items that make up the corresponding section for the ith observation unit; x_{min} It is the minimum value observed of the sum of the rating granted for the items that make up the corresponding section for the ith observation unit; $x_{máx}$ It is the minimum value observed of the sum of the rating granted for the items that make up the corresponding section for the ith observation unit.

Based on these results, the competitiveness index (IndComp) is obtained as the weighted average of the marketing, innovation and finance indexes, by means of the expression:

$$IndComp_i = (0.35)\ IndMer_i + (0.35)\ IndInnov_i + (0.3)\ IndFnz_i \qquad (3)$$

The weights assigned to the marketing, innovation and finance factors are the result of the analysis of the literature, the opinion of the owners, and the representatives of the livestock associations, with respect to the relative importance of said factors in the competitiveness of the production units. As can be seen, the value reflects a similar importance for the three factors with a greater relative importance of marketing and innovation, with respect to finance.

Nine subthemes based on the same number of reagent subgroups (three for each section of the survey) were previously established to identify the relationship between the sub-themes and the competitiveness index. For each subtheme, an indicator was constructed from the corresponding subgroup of reagents using the threshold method. The subthemes and indicators by section are the following:

- Marketing:
  - Market positioning.
  - Knowledge of the competition.
  - Customer satisfaction.
- Innovation:
  - Innovation in processes.
  - Innovation in products.
  - Investigation and development.
- Finance:
  - Use of information.
  - Cost effectiveness.
  - Sources of financing.

To analyze the relationship between subtopics and the competitiveness index, three models of multiple linear regression were performed, reviewing in addition to compliance with the assumptions of the constructed models, the standardized regression coefficients and the p-values associated with said coefficients in said models. The general results of the analyses are presented in **Table 6**.

In accordance with the above, considering the value of the standardized regression coefficients as a measure of the relative importance that the aspects of each section (marketing, innovation and finance) have in relation to the competitiveness of the observation units, as well as the values p of the tests of statistical significance for the regression coefficients under study, the results are the following.

In relation to marketing, the aspects most related to competitiveness are market positioning and customer satisfaction, which coincides with [26–28] who consider the competitiveness factor to include these variables as the real generators of competitiveness. Regarding innovation, the most closely related aspects are innovation in products and innovation in processes; this coincides with what was pointed out by [21], who states that the variables of innovation of process and innovation of product are indispensable for the competitiveness of the organizations. Finally, regarding finances, the most closely related aspects are the sources of financing, the use of financial information and profitability; this coincides with principles established by [31, 34].

Concept	Marketing	Innovation	Finance
Model	$y = 0.378\,x_1 + 0.152\,x_2 + 0.329$ $x_3 + 1.829$	$y = 0.306\,x_1 + 0.578$ $x_2 + 0.001\,x_3 + 7.798$	$y = 0.269\,x_1 + 0.515\,x_2 + 0.461$ $x_3 - 7.609$
Standardized coefficient B1	0.463	0.334	0.328
Standardized coefficient B2	0.166	0.671	0.309
Standardized coefficient B3	0.375	0.001	0.408
R^2 adjusted	0.956 (95.6%)	0.973 (97.3%)	0.943 (94.3%)
Durbin Watson coefficient	2.081	2.201	1.545
P value (ANOVA)	0.000	0.000	0.000
P value (B1)	0.006	0.001	0.003
P value (B2)	0.220	0.000	0.000
P value (B3)	0.007	0.988	0.000
P values (B0)	0.481	0.000	0.058
P value of the test of Kolmogorov-Smirnov	0.995	0.996	0.960
Homoscedasticity	ok	ok	ok

Source: Own elaboration based on research data.

Table 6. Results of multiple linear regression analysis.

The other aspects were not statistically significant in relation to the built models, that is, their relative importance is minimal.

3. Conclusions and recommendations

3.1. Conclusions

The population studied was made up of 18 cattle ranches in the municipality of Tizimín (60%), 5 cattle ranches in the municipality of Panabá (16.7%), 3 in the municipality of Sucilá (10%) and the rest in the municipalities of Buctzotz, Cenotillo, Dzilam González and Sotuta, each of these, with only one ranch.

Ranching operations are, on the average, 31 years old. They have an average of 27 full-time workers working in them, with an average of 1120 head of cattle and a territorial extension of 1306 ha. It was found that the owners are on average 57 years of age.

The competitiveness index model (IndComp) is obtained as the weighted average of the marketing, innovation and finance indexes.

The finance indicator has the lowest maximum value as compared to the other two indicators related to marketing and innovation and the competitiveness index itself.

The competitiveness of most of the observation units at a medium level could be qualified.

There is a statistically significant negative correlation with the years of foundation and the age of the owner; that is, it seems that the seniority of the ranch or greater age of the owner is associated with lower competitiveness. On the other hand, a larger-sized observation unit (according to the heads of livestock or hectares it has) is more competitive. The generation of the competitiveness index as well as the importance of the factors analyzed in the study (finance, marketing and innovation), allows all those involved in the sector to develop strategies to boost their competitiveness.

3.2. Recommendations

It will be necessary to have qualified workers in order to use the most sophisticated technology in the breeding and fattening of cattle. Bearing in mind that there are many small cattle producers that produce independently of the largest cattle farmers, the smaller producers should consider working together in order to create outsourcing alliances to obtain cost advantages in the acquisition of raw material.

Cattle meat producers could benefit more from production if they could further exploit economies of scale in the production and distribution of new food products. They could also increase the production of high-end products. Finally, they should focus the growth of their external sales to the countries of high consumption and high growth and with which there are trade agreements, such as China and Vietnam.

Farmers and related industries should invest in research in order to develop local technology, in relation to biotechnology as well as equipment. Although some progress has been made in this regard, there is an opportunity to develop the machinery that can be tested and improved locally. When the results are positive, the machinery can be easily exported later to other beef producers in the world. The development of more suppliers and support for industries would be very beneficial, as it increases competition and innovation among suppliers. This gives companies more opportunities to improve costs.

It is necessary to improve local competition and cooperation abroad. Because there are high fixed costs to enter new world markets, strategic alliances could be made between producers entering foreign markets.

Some of the limitations that could be mentioned are the context in which it can be applicable, as well as the lack of vision and the ingrained organizational culture that hinders innovation.

As a contribution for future studies, this work offers a strategic model and a methodology to boost competitiveness and the generation of added value. However, there could be, in addition to the factors analyzed in this study, other factors that could have an important effect on competitiveness of the sector. This study can also be replicated in other states to identify the competitiveness index of the livestock sector as well as in other sectors to assess their competitiveness. In Mexico, there are few studies related to the generation of the competitiveness index of the different sectors. In the specific case of the beef sector, the information obtained is generated by government entities such as SAGARPA, the Ministry of Economy as well as local secretariats, which are based on data on production, exports, and so on. This information is important, but the lack of an index of competitiveness of the different productive sectors of each federative entity impedes comparison among the sectors in order to develop strategies to boost their competitiveness.

Author details

Antonio Emmanuel Perez Brito*, Teresa de Jesus Espinosa Atoche and
Karla Patricia Quintal Gordillo

*Address all correspondence to: antonio.perez@correo.uady.mx

Autonomous University of Yucatan, Yucatan, Mexico

References

[1] Organización para la Cooperación y el Desarrollo Económico (OCDE, 2009). Información Básica del Sector Agropecuario, Subregión Norte de America Latina y el Caribe. Available at: http://www.oecd.org/pages/0,3417,es_36288966_36288120_1_1_1_1_1,0 [Accessed: April 18, 2018]

[2] Organización de las Naciones Unidas para la Agricultura y la Alimentación (FAO, 2013). El Estado Mundial de la Agricultura y la Alimentación. Available at: http://www.fao.org/docrep/018/i3300e/i3300e00.htm. [Accessed: April 20, 2018]

[3] González E. La Sanidad y el Estado Sanitario del Hato Nacional de Bovinos para Carne. México: CONASA; 2006. 75 p

[4] Secretaría de Agricultura, Ganadería, Desarrollo Rural, Pesca y Alimentación (SAGARPA). Situación actual y Perspectivas de la producción de carne bovino en México. 2011. Available at: http://www.ipcva.com.ar/files/mexico.pdf [Accessed: April 15, 2018]

[5] Instituto Nacional de Estadística y Geografía, Sistema de Cuentas Nacionales de México, México. XIII Censo General de Población y Vivienda 2010. 2010. Available at: http://www.inegi.org.mx/est/contenidos/proyectos/ccpv/cpv2010/presentacion. [Accessed: March 22, 2018]

[6] Anderson S, Santos J, Boden R, Wadsworth J. Characterization of Cattle Production Systems in the State of Yucatan. Dual Purpose Cattle Production Research, vol. 40. México: Fundación Internacional para la Ciencia; 2012. pp. 187-192

[7] Hernández J, Rebollar S, González F, Guzmán E, Albarrán P, García M. La cadena productiva de ganado bovino en el sur del estado de México, México. Revista Mexicana de Agronegocios. 2011;29:672-680

[8] Martínez V, Santos J, Montes R. Función de producción de la ganadería de doble propósito de la zona oriente del estado de Yucatán. México. Técnica Pecuaria en México. 2012;40:187-192

[9] Fava M, Canto F, Melo M. Competitiveness of Brazilian beef chain, vol. 50. Brasil: IFAMA; 2012. pp. 1-13

[10] Vera J, Ganga F. Los Clústers Industriales: Precisión Conceptual y Desarrollo Teórico, vol. 20. Colombia: Cuadernos de Administración; 2007. pp. 303-323

[11] Secretaría de Economía (SE). Sectores Agropecuarios. 2009. Available at: http//:www.economia.gob.mx [Accessed: February 22, 2018]

[12] Dussauge P, Hart S, Ramanantsoa B. Strategic Technology Management. Inglaterra: John Wiley &Sons Ltd; 1992. 93 p

[13] Lewis W, Gersbach H, Jansen T, Sakate K. The Secret to Competitiveness. Estados Unidos. The Mc Kinsey Quarterly. 1993;1:1-8

[14] Bradenburguer A, Nalebuff B. Competencia. Colombia: Grupo Editorial Norma; 1996. 15 p

[15] Duncan J, Ginter M, Swayne L. Competitive Advantage and Internal Organization Assessment. Estados Unidos. Academy of Management Executive. 1998;3:6-17. DOI: 10.5465/ame.1998.1109046

[16] Rueda I, Simón N. Globalización y competitividad. La Industria Siderúrgica ubicada en México. México: Editorial Porrúa; 2002. 85 p

[17] Blunck F. What is competitiveness? Estados Unidos. Competitiveness Summer School. 2006;**74**:1-32

[18] Perea J, Rivas L. Estrategias competitivas para los productores cafetaleros de la región de Cordova, Veracruz. México. Revista de la Facultad de Contaduría y Administración de la UNAM. 2008;**24**:9-33

[19] Pisano G, Shih W. Restoring American Competitiveness. Estados Unidos. Harvard Business Review. 2009;**80**:2-14. DOI: 10.1080/09692290.2012.756414

[20] Malhotra V, Manyika J. Five misconceptions about the productivity. Estados Unidos. The Mc Kinsey Quarterly. 2011;**15**:1-3

[21] Porter M. The Competitive Advantage of Nations. Estados Unidos: Harvard Business Press; 1990. 76 p

[22] Schroeder, R. Administración de operaciones. México: Editorial Mc Graw Hill; 1992. 15 p

[23] Foro Ecónomico Mundial. Índice de Competitividad Global 2011-2012 [The Global Competitiveness Report 2011-2012]. 2012; 389513-14. Available at: www3.weforum. org [Accessed: March 30, 2018]

[24] Ramaswamy V, Gatignon H, Reibstein D. Competitive marketing behavior in industrial markets. Journal of Marketing. 1994;**58**:45-55. DOI: 10.2307/1252268

[25] Galán J, Vecino J. Las Fuentes de Rentabilidad de las Empresas. Revista Europea de Dirección y Economía de la Empresa. 1997;**1**(6):21-36

[26] Stanton W, Etzel M, Walker B. Fundamentos de Marketing. México: Mc Graw Hill; 2000. 33 p

[27] Jeffrey H, Caron J. Fundamentos de Dirección Estratégica. España: Thompson editores; 2002. 21 p

[28] Fischer L, Espejo J. Mercadotecnia. México: McGraw Hill; 2004. 43 p

[29] Gitman L. Fundamentos de Administración Financiera. México: Editorial Harla; 1986. 11 p

[30] David F. Conceptos de Administración Estratégica. México: Pearson Editores; 2003. 29 p

[31] Birley S, Westhead P. Growth and Performance Contrasts between Types of Small Firms. Strategic Management Journal. 1990;**11**:535-557. DOI: 10.1002/smj.4250110705

[32] Bantel K, Jackson S. Top management and innovations in banking: Does the composition of the top team make the difference. Strategic Management Journal. 1989;**10**:107-124. DOI: 10.1002/smj.4250100709

[33] Norburn D, Birley S. The top management team and corporate performance. Strategic Management Journal. 1988;**9**:225-237. DOI: 10.1002/smj.4250090303

[34] Sallenave J. La gerencia integral. Colombia: Grupo Editorial Norma; 1994. 22 p

[35] Unión Ganadera Regional del Oriente de Yucatán (UGROY). Registros de Socios 2013. México. 2014. 12 p

[36] Olivares A, Coronado J. Liderazgo y Competitividad. México: Pearson; 2013. 15 p

[37] Thompson B, Larry D. Factor analytic evidence for the construct validity of scores: A historical overview and some guidelines. Educational and Psychological Measurement. 1996;**56**:197-208. DOI: 10.1177/0013164496056002001

[38] Cerny C, Kaiser H. A study of a measure of samping adequacy for factor-analytic correlation matrices. Multivariate Behavioral Research. 1977;**12**:43-47. DOI: 10.1207/s15327906mbr1201_3

[39] Anderson D, Sweeney D, Williams T. Estadística para Administración y Economía. México: Cengaje Learning; 2008. 41 p

[40] Conover W. Practical nonparametric statistics. Estados Unidos: John Wiley & Sons; 1980. 92 p

[41] Pengfei N. Urban Competitiveness in China. China: Social Sciencie Academic Press; 2006. 19 p

Bovine Feed Manipulation, Enhancement of Conjugated Linoleic Acid and Its Bioavailability

Nazir Ahmad, Muhammad Kamran Khan, Muhammad Imran,
Muhammad Nadeem Suleman and Sufyan Afzal

Additional information is available at the end of the chapter

http://dx.doi.org/10.5772/intechopen.79306

Abstract

Diet is a pivotal contributing factor to the onset and progression of some chronic ailments nowadays. The conjugated linoleic acid (CLA), a bioactive component of ruminant fat, introduces more elucidates what we know polyunsaturated fats and diseases. CLA, a mixture of isomers c9, t11 and t10, c12, is the most abundant ranging from 80 to 90% of total CLA isomers and account for most known health benefits. Dairy milk and meat are the major dietary sources of CLA, and its concentration is of great interest to human health. The biofunctionalities of CLA from enriched dairy products are major attributes in the context of a substance present in our everyday diet. Thus, dietary modifications in animal feed, synthetic and microbial production have been made to increase CLA intake to enhance its clinical manifestations. However, the bioavailability and distribution of enriched or supplemented CLA has not been fully elucidated because of its response variation in different animal models. This chapter deals with different dietary sources, availability, enhancement of CLA in dairy products and its positive manifestation against different maladies. In conclusion, it is feasible to produce CLA-enriched dairy products with acceptable storage and sensory characteristics while deriving its nutritional benefits.

Keywords: feed manipulation, essential fatty acids, conjugated linoleic acid, enhancement, bioavailability

1. Introduction

The consumption of dietary fat and fatty acids is still the prominent focusing on human nutrition and health research. This continuing trend in research not only leads to classify fat as saturated, unsaturated, monounsaturated, polyunsaturated and omega fatty acids but also the essential role of fairly small and relatively specific fatty acid called, conjugated linoleic acid (CLA). CLA is a mixture of isomers that are characterized by the presence of conjugated dienes on different geometric positions coming from ruminant to human diet primarily in meat and milk products [1]. The promising health effects of CLA are the major interest of research in fatty acids. CLA from dairy sources has predominant isomers such as c9, t11 and t10, c12 and has shown biological effects against modern nutritional disorders [2]. These dairy products with natural CLA concentration ranging from 0.34 to 1.07 g/100 g fat in milk and 0.12 to 0.68 g/100 g fat in meat [3, 4] but this CLA concentration is not sufficient to meet daily requirement (1.5 to 3.5 g/day) of human being [5, 6].

To meet the recommended daily CLA intake, production and sale of meat and milk products supplemented and/or enrichment with essential fatty acids, particularly CLA has increased drastically from the late 1990s due to its biofunctionalities. Several efforts have been made to increase the concentration of CLA in these dairy products for pronounced health effects. In this context, the feeding practices of dairy animals let them to change nutrients concentration, particularly the fatty acids composition in its milk and meat and its products. However, these bio-enriched dairy products do not differ in their nutrient composition as compared to the conventional foods. Animal diet modifications result in change of amount of trans fatty acids, unsaturated fatty acids, ratio of 3:6 omega fatty acids but most pronounced difference was observed in concentration of CLA while feeding on grain supplemented diet as compared to pastures diet [7, 8].

To date, there is a lot of scientific literature on animal feedings practices and effects of CLA on human health but there are relatively very few studies on the bioavailability of CLA from dairy products and more precisely, the bioavailability of CLA from these naturally bio-fortified dairy products needs to be fully explored. It is generally considered that c-9, t-11 CLA from dairy products and animal meat accounts of 90 and 75%, respectively, while plant oils have less than 50% c-9, t-1I CLA isomer in total CLA. It formulated as biologically active form that tended to become less active in processed dairy and meats products [1]. Furthermore, the comparative human health effect of CLA products from dairy products remains inconclusive. Most of the previous studies were conducted on animals, and secondly, in most of these studies, synthetic mixtures of CLA supplement were used that do not mimic the similar functions as CLA from natural food sources possess and do not confound differently with potential risk factors [9]. To our knowledge, this is the first manuscript to discuss the bioavailability of CLA from dairy products obtained by ruminant diets modification and chemically synthesized CLA.

1.1. Biosynthesis of CLA

The biosynthesis of CLA in ruminants depends on content of diet and microbial and enzymatic action. CLA isomers produce either in rumen or in the intestine as shown in **Figure 1**. For example, the major isomers of CLA, cis-9, trans-11 CLA is produced in rumen from dietary linoleic and linolenic acids by microbial biohydrogenation [10, 11]. The major pathway in the biosynthesis of cis-9, trans-11 CLA in cow's milk is the biohydrogenation and desaturation. After microbial biohydrogenation of cis-9, trans-11, it is further bio-hydrogenated to *trans*-11-octadecenoic acid if not absorbed directly. Bioconversion of trans-vaccenic acid to cis-9, trans-11 CLA is occurred with the help of stearoyl-CoA desaturase action in ruminants [12, 13]. The presence of *trans*-10, *cis*-12 in ruminant's milk indicates that *cis*-9, *trans*-11 CLA and *trans*-10, *cis*-12 CLA have been converted to *trans*-10-octadecenoic acid via biohydrogenation in rumen. But due to lack of delta 12 desaturase, mammal could not desaturate *trans*-10-octadec-enoic acid back to *trans*-10, *cis*-12 CLA depositing *trans*-10, *cis*-12 CLA in their tissues [12, 14].

1.2. CLA bio-fortification through diet manipulation

The presence of CLA intrigues the researchers to look at the possible ways of increasing the concentration of CLA in ruminant's milk, meat and other dairy products for its positive health promising functionalities. These products are the principle source of nutrients, minerals and vitamins. Among these, dairy milk is the major dietary source with highest concentration of CLA. All ruminants under normal physiological conditions produce only 0.2–2.0% CLA of total tissue or milk fat [16, 17]. While the consumption of 120 g beef fat having CLA concentra-tions from 1.2 to 12.5 mg/g of fat accounts for total recommended daily intake of 1.5 to 3.5 g of CLA [5, 6]. This naturally low level of CLA makes very difficult to consume large quantity of fat to meet daily-recommended intake of CLA. Thus, several interventions have been made to enhance CLA concentration on milk and meat. For this purpose, different animals, their breeds, diet manipulations, commercial/synthetic CLA production, use of different strains of microbes have been used as strategies. Dietary manipulation is one of the approaches to increase natural production and enhancement of CLA in dairy products [18].

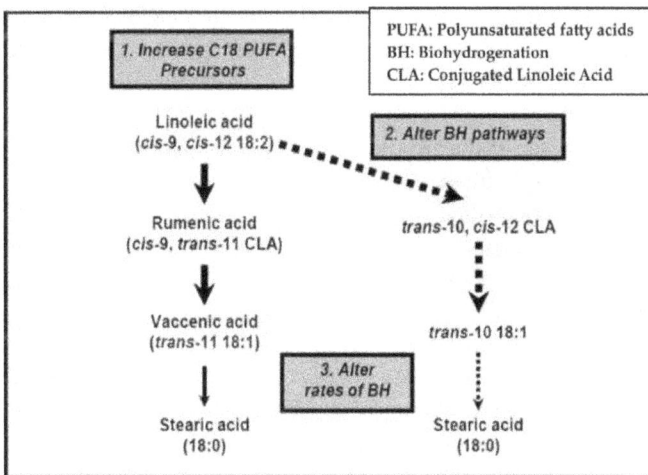

Figure 1. Schematic representation of linoleic acid in ruminants under normal (left side) and diet-induced milk fat formation (right side) [15].

1.3. Bio-fortified CLA in bovine's milk

Different diet manipulations, seasonal effects and farm characteristics (e.g., organic vs. traditional) have been used to enhance CLA concentration in milk of cow and buffalo. The diet-manipulating strategies and their effects on CLA enhancement in milk have been summarized in **Table 1**. It was observed the dietary substrates of CLA in animal feed results result in an increase of CLA in milk, most variation in cow milk [19–21]. It has been shown that the concentration of milk CLA is as result of interaction between the diet composition and fatty acid profile of diet supplement. This complex interaction greatly influences greatly the biohydrogenation of supplemented fat in rumen and the formation of CLA. For example, Holstein cow fed with high concentrate and forage at the ratio of 65:35 along with 5 g/100 g dry matter of sunflower oil, 5 g/100 g linseed oil or 2.5 g/100 g fish oil drained out greater CLA in milk as compared to control without fat supplementation. The cow fed on sunflower oil drained out greater total CLA (8.3 g/day vs. 4.0 g/day) as compared to feed consist of fish oil while linseed oil feeding results in 6.9 g/day of total CLA. The cis9, trans11-CLA (0.22 g/100 g total fatty acids) was higher in case of feeding on sunflower oil compared to linseed oil (0.13 g/100 g) and fish oil (0.06 g/100 g) [22]. Another study conducted to evaluate the effects of sunflower oil in dairy rations for vaccenic (trans-11-18:1) and rumenic acids (cis-9, trans-11-18:2) production in milk, the animal were fed with forage and concentrate of barley/alfalfa/hay barley-alfalfa-hay silage and corn/barley grain. They reported that there was linear increase in total trans-18:1 (5.2, 9.1, 14.1, and 21.3%) and total CLA (0.7, 1.9, 2.4, and 3.9%), respectively. The rumenic acid concentration also increased in linear pattern from 0.43, 1.5, 1.9, and 3.4% for 10 days feeding period and 0.42, 2.15, 2.09, and 2.78% for 38 days feeding period, respectively. Rumenic acid increased from 66 to 85% using sunflower, linseed and fish oil supplement in cow's feed. CLA enhancement of 4.5-fold by feeding 3% sunflower, oil/fish oil appears to be most promising in trans-11-18:1 and cis-9, trans-11-18:2. While total saturated fatty acids declined to 18%. A good and healthy composition of fatty acids including 4% vaccenic and 2% rumenic acids was achieved by feeding 3% sunflower oil and 0.5% fish oil in animal diet dry matter [23, 24]. Bell et al. adopted three dietary strategies to enhance the flow of CLA in cow milk. The Holstein cows were fed for 2 weeks with control diet of forage and dry matter while 6%, monensin, safflower and safflower oil as experimental diet. The cis-9, trans-11 CLA in milk increased from 0.45 to 5.15% of total fatty acids for control or experimental diet. Furthermore, the addition of vitamin E supplementation resulted in retained the CLA content in milk of cow [25]. The high corn and corn silage dietary feeding strategy was also observed in increase of cow milk from 3.8 and 3.9 mg/g total fatty acids, respectively. The Alfalfa hay and concentrates replacing all pasture by one-third, two-thirds resulted in increase of milk CLA to 8.9, 14.3, and 22.1 mg/g. Grazing pasture only led to 500% more CLA as compared to feeding on typical dairy diets. Gairn with alfalfa with fish oil and monensin supplement resulted in 6.8 mg/g of milk total fatty acids [14]. Beside fatty acids dietary modification, other diet components modification also resulted in increase the concentration of cow milk CLA. For example, studies of Morales et al. have shown that tannin diet contents can modify the milk CLA concentration. The tannin supplementation in feeding cow diet cow feed affects the microfloura of rumen resulting in unsaturated fatty acids biohydrogenation and hence influencing linolenic acid (c9, c12, c15–18:3), vaccenic acid (t11–18:1) and rumenic acid (c9, t11–18:2) [26]. Tyagi studied the effects of green fodder feeding on CLA in milk fat of buffaloes. There was and reported that there was

Feed type	Feed specialty	CLA (control)	CLA (treatment)	Reference
Grass hay, concentrates	Fish oil	0.72 mg/g	2.83 mg/g	[30]
Grass hay, concentrates	Sunflower oil and wheat starch	0.72 mg/g	1.33 mg/g	[30]
Hay forage, concentrate	CLA (38%) + EPA + DHA 36.5% and humic-mineral carrier	2.33 mg/g	2.78 mg/g	[31]
Egyptian clover, sorghum forage	Rice straw	0.433 mg/g	1.0.4 mg/g	[32]
Egyptian clover, sorghum forage	*Pleurotus ostreatus*	0.27 mg/g	0.80 mg/g	[32]
Corn silage, 27.7% dietary starch	Fish oil (0.80%)	0.48 mg/g fat	0.76 mg/g fat	[33]
Forage, concentrate, palm oil (300 g/day)	Linseed oil (300 g/day)	0.82 mg/g fat	1.90 mg/g fat	[34]
Forage, concentrate, palm oil (300 g/day)	Top dressed whole linseed (688 g/day)	0.82 mg/g fat	2.05 mg/g fat	[34]
Concentrate	Pasture and extruded soybeans	15.4 percentage FA	24.2 percentage FA	[35]
Alfalfa, corn silage, concentrate	Fish oil (2%)	2.86 mg/g fat	3.14 mg/g fat	[36]
Alfalfa, corn silage, concentrate	Canola oil + fish oil (1:1)	2.86 mg/g fat	3.32 mg/g fat	[36]
Alfalfa, corn silage, concentrate	Canola oil (2%)	2.86 mg/g fat	3.16 mg/g fat	[36]
Concentrate, maize ground, soybean, cane molasses, alfalfa	Whole cottonseed	7.59 percentage FA	9.36 percentage FA	[22]
Alfalfa hay forage	Sunflower oil	0.65 g/100 g fatty acids	0.80 g/100 g fatty acids	[37]
Alfalfa hay forage	Hydrogenated palm oil	0.65 g/100 g fatty acids	0.71 g/100 g fatty acids	[37]
Indoor concentrate	Pasture	4.3 mg/g fat	6.80 mg/g fat	[38]
Grass forage	Sunflower oil (255 g/day)	1.76 mg/g fat	1.87 mg/g fat	[39]
Grass forage	Sunflower oil: fish oil (255:52.5 g/day)	1.76 mg/g fat	2.36 mg/g fat	[39]
Grass forage	Fish oil (105 g/day)	1.76 mg/g fat	2.16 mg/g fat	[39]
Animal fat (400 g)	Fish oil: sunflower oil (100 g:300 g)	2.02 mg/g fat	3.41 mg/g fat	[40]
Typical indoor concentrate	Pasture + sunflower oil (100 g/kg.day)	0.46 mg/g fat	2.22 mg/g fat	[41]
Wheat straw, concentrate	Sunflower seed supplemented (11.2%)	0.54 mg/g fat	2.0 mg/g fat	[23]

Feed type	Feed specialty	CLA (control)	CLA (treatment)	Reference
Corn silage-based rations	Fish oil (45 g) + sunflower oil (45 g)	0.50 mg/g fat	3.47 mg/g fat	[42]
Hay supplemented with tallow	Fresh forage supplemented with tallow	0.93 mg/g fat	1.07 mg/g fat	[43]
Hay supplemented with tallow	Fresh forage + ground solin seed	0.93 mg/g fat	1.30 mg/g fat	[43]
Concentrate (50%), corn silage (25%), alfalfa hay (25%)	Fish oil (0.5%)	0.33 mg/g fat	0.47 mg/g fat	[44]
Concentrate (50%), corn silage (25%), alfalfa hay (25%)	Soybean oil (2.5%)	0.33 mg/g fat	0.79 mg/g fat	[44]
Concentrate (50%), corn silage (25%), alfalfa hay (25%)	Fish oil: soybean oil (0.5%:2%)	0.33 mg/g fat	1.39 mg/g fat	[44]
Grass silage	Fish oil	0.2–0.6 mg/g fat	1.5–2.7 mg/g fat	[45]
Grass silage	Fish oil	0.2–0.6 mg/g fat	1.5–2.7 mg/g fat	[45]
Forage and grain (TMR)	Pasture feeding	3.8 g/100 g fatty acids	22.1 g/100 g fatty acids	[14]
Dry matter with blood meal, feather meal and corn gluten	Sunflower oil (53 g/kg)	3.55 g/100 g fatty acids	24.4 g/100 g fatty acids	[46]
Dry matter with blood meal, feather meal and corn gluten	Linseed oil (53 g/kg)	3.55 g/100 g fatty acids	16.7 g/100 g fatty acids	[46]
Dry matter with blood meal, feather meal and corn gluten	Peanut oil (53 g/kg)	3.55 g/100 g fatty acids	13.3 g/100 g fatty acids	[46]
DM + 4% calcium salts	Canola oil	3.5 g/100 g fatty acids	13.0 g/100 g fatty acids	[47]
DM + 4% calcium salts	Soybean oil	3.5 g/100 g fatty acids	22.0 g/100 g fatty acids	[47]
DM + 4% calcium salts	Linseed oil	3.5 g/100 g fatty acids	19.0 g/100 g fatty acids	[47]

CLA represents two major CLA isomers of C18:2 cis-9, trans-11 and trans-10, cis-12 isomer, TMR: total mixed ration, DM: dry matter, FA: fatty acid.

Table 1. Effect of feed modification on CLA content in bovine's milk.

no change in milk composition of buffaloes with respect to dietary treatments while 310% increase in CLA contents were increased was observed by feeding buffalo on green fodder [27]. The starch diet containing high proportions of polyunsaturated fatty acid promotes shifts in biohydrogenation mechanism, which results in major intermediate trans isomers [28, 29].

Griinari et al. made an attempt by modifying the endogenous activity of D9-desaturase, which involves in synthesis of CLA from trans-11 18:1 in ruminal biohydrogenation [12]. They observed that infusion of trans-11 18:1 resulted in a 31% increase of concentration of cis-9, trans-11 CLA in milk fat. While induction of D9-desaturase inhibitor in cow abdomen resulted in a 45% decrease of 45% in the concentration of CLA. Overall, they concluded that endogenous synthesis of CLA is the primary source of milk CLA in ruminants.

1.4. Bio-fortified CLA in bovine's meat

Recent studies on different feed resources and their influence on meat quality in the term of CLA from small ruminants showed that CLA content in meat would be increased due to chopped cactus cladodes feeding to animals. The oil supplementation in all forms of safflower soybean, sunflower, linseed and fish oil results in enhancement of CLA contents in meat of small as well as large ruminants. Furthermore, reducing anti-nutritional components in above oil sources leads to more enhancements in CLA content of meat in all ruminants [48–54]. For example, a very recent study by Fiorentini et al. reported that feeding palm oil, linseed oil, soybean grain or protected fat result in increased the meat CLA contents from 0.29 to 0.67 mg/100-gram fatty acid, respectively in Nellore steers [53]. While feeding 4.5% linseed, sunflower, or soybean enhances meat CLA content to 0.47, 0.52 and 0.54 mg/100 g fatty in Holstein Friesian bulls. Similar CLA enhancement was observed when Nellore steer were fed with cottonseed at different proportion to dry matter. However, the reducing anti-nutritional contents of linseed, soybean or sunflower, and so on further led to enhance the CLA contents from 0.73 mg/100 g to 0.91 mg/100 g fatty acid in meat [55]. Joele et al. reported that 11% supplementation of coconut or 15% palm cake enhanced 7.98 and 4.98% of CLA contents, respectively, in buffalo Red Norte meet [52]. Fish oil supplementation in concentrate-based diet of Charolais steer results in enhancement of meat CLA content to 0.57% to total fatty acids [56]. Similarly, pasture grazing of small as well as large ruminants enhances the CLA content of meat. More notably, pasture grazing leads to CLA substantial increase as a proportion of total fatty acids and is more available in the form of edible fat as compared to the CLA concentration present in raw meat. This pasturing strategy also leads to reduced total fat contents in raw meat as well as product. On the other shrubs that are rich in vitamin E, protect myoglobin from oxidation and grazing saltbush (*Atriplex* spp.), preserves lamb meat color stability, while linoleic acid contents may increase in meat fat by adding olive cake silage in ewe or lamb diets, respectively. Grazing on some novel pasture species, such as *Cichorium intybus*, *Chrisantemum coronarium*, and *Galium verum* enhanced the appearance of terpenes in goat and sheep meat. Although the dietary factors contribute significantly in the increase of CLA content in milk and meat but only marginal increases in meat is observed as compared to milk. The possible mechanisms and synthesis pathway of CLA may be different according to organ site. Furthermore, other related factors regulating the synthesis of CLA in the rumen muscles and mammary glands are poorly understood [57, 58]. **Table 2** shows the different strategies with increase CLA contents in meat of bovine.

1.5. Bio-fortified CLA milk's cheese and butter

Most of the studies show that the milk processing and cooking do not influence the CLA concentration in milk by products like such as cheese, butter, and ice cream, and so on. The cheese

Breed	CLA enhancing diet	CLA content	References
Nellore steers	Palm oil	0.29 mg/g fat	[53]
Nellore steers	Linseed oil	0.67 mg/g fat	[53]
Nellore steers	Protected fat	0.39 mg/g fat	[53]
Nellore steers	Soybean grains	0.37 mg/g fat	[53]
Steers	Pasture and extruded soybeans	25.0 g/100 g fatty acids	[35]
Rubia Gallega calves	4.5% Linseed	0.47 mg/g fat	[59]
Rubia Gallega calves	4.5% Sunflower	0.52 mg/g fat	[59]
Rubia Gallega calves	4.5% Soybean	0.54 mg/g fat	[59]
Nellore steers	Cottonseed (14.35 kg/100 kg DM)	0.28 mg/g fat	[48]
Nellore steers	Cottonseed (27.51 kg/100 kg DM)	0.29 mg/g fat	[48]
Nellore steers	Cottonseed (34.09 kg/100 kg DM)	0.24 mg/g fat	[48]
Yearling steers	Flax seed oil	0.76 mg/g fat	[49]
Yearling steers	Sunflower seed oil	0.85 mg/g fat	[49]
Yearling steers	Flax seed oil	0.79 mg/g fat	[49]
Yearling steers	Sunflower seed oil	0.86 mg/g fat	[49]
Charolais × Saler steers	Extruded linseed 4%	0.72 mg/g fat	[55]
Charolais cows	Extruded linseed 4%	0.40 mg/g fat	[55]
Holstein cows	Extruded linseed 4%	0.99 mg/g fat	[55]
Charolais bulls	Extruded linseed 4%	0.91 mg/g fat	[55]
German Holstein, bulls	Pasture	17 g/100 g fatty acids	[60]
German Simmental, bulls	Pasture	12 g/100 g fatty acids	[60]
Wagyu x Limousin, steers	whole concentrate	0.12 mg/g fat	[5]
Charolais steers	Grass silage	35 g/100 g fatty acids	[61]
Holstein calves	Megalac	15·9 g/100 g fatty acids	[62]
Holstein calves	Protected lipid supplement	14·5 g/100 g fatty acids	[62]
Holstein calves	Protected lipid supplement	10.1 g/100 g fatty acids	[62]
Angus × Hereford	Finishing diet + soy oil	0.28 mg/g fat	[63]
Limousin, steers	Sunflower oil	134 g/100 g fatty acids	[64]
Angus steers	Concentrate + soy oil (6%)	0.34 mg/g fat	[65]
Angus steers	Concentrate + extruded soybean	0.73 mg/g fat	[66]
Angus crossbred steers	Whole pasture	1.5 mg/g fat	[67]
Charolais steers	Grass based + concentrate	1.1 mg/g fat	[68]
Wagyu crossbred	Barley-based diet	1.7 mg/FA	[69]
Charolais steers	Grass silage whole linseed	36 g/100 g fatty acids	[56]

Breed	CLA enhancing diet	CLA content	References
Charolais steers	Concentrate based + linseed	0.80 mg/g fat	[56]
Holstein claves	53 g/kg Sunflower oil	24.4 g/100 g fatty acids	[46]

CLA represents two major CLA isomers of C18:2 cis-9, trans-11 and trans-10, cis-12 isomer, TMR: total mixed ration, DM: dry matter, FA: fatty acid.

Table 2. Effect of diet modification on CLA content in bovine's meat.

prepared from milk produced by diet supplementing with soybean, extruded soybean, soybean, and so on in cows, soybean oils, extruded soybean, olive oil and palm oils, linseed and extruded linseed, and flaxseed meal, flaxseed oil, castor oil and soybean, and so on in goats resulted in stable CLA content [31, 70–72]. For example, the milk cheese prepared using milk from cows fed extruded soybeans and cottonseed shows the same concentration of CLA in cheese as it was present in milk [73]. Fish oil supplement in all ruminants also resulted shows in enhancement of CLA content cheese from milk used for cheese preparation. Furthermore, the CLA enhancement effects were more predominant when starter culture was used in cheese manufacturing process [74, 75]. The pasture grazing strategy is also significant to enhance the CLA contents in cheese and butter. Other reports have shown that the quality and composition of sheep and goat milk influenced by farming and feeding systems while comparing three feeding systems based on natural pasture in the plain, on mountains and on hills for goats. Thus, milk yield was shown to be lower to some extent on mountain pasture while percentages of PUFA, protein and fat contents were high. Therefore, the terpenes were more abundant in goat milk. On the other hand, milk was richer in CLA at an early stage of natural pasture grazing. Simultaneously, the milk products like cheese, butter and ice cream prepared from goat milk produced by feeding on diet enriched with castor, sesame and faveleira vegetable oils showed enhance CLA content in these products [72, 76, 77]. **Table 3** shows the summarized results of different dietary manipulation strategies to enhance CLA contents in cheeses and butters.

1.6. Enrichment of CLA

1.6.1. Commercial/synthetic CLA

The low percentage rate of CLA conversion by ruminants was accounting as very small in total percentage of fat and oil as dietary sources. The highly bioactive importance of CLA derived the focus to develop commercial CLA. Several methods were developed by using a series of acids and bases reactions to convert polyunsaturated oils to CLA. The earlier attempt to produce commercial CLA resulted in unnatural ratios of CLA isomers. The first successful attempt to develop drying oil from linolenic acid oils using monohydric and polyhydric solution with addition of numerous alkalis as catalysts. Later, another development, a modification was made by the use of water and steam to achieve a required temperature to conjugate unsaturated fatty acids. Moreover, the successive addition of mineral acid led to the successful development of free conjugated fatty acids production method [80, 81]. Christie et al. first time reported to develop a CLA product by alkaline water isomerization (KOH and NaOH catalyst at temperature > 280°C) which have all 8, 10: 9, 11: 10, 12: 11,13 trans and cis CLA

CLA enhancing feed	CLA content	Reference
Pasture + extruded soybean	1.4 g/100 g fatty acid	[16]
Whole pasture	1.5 g/100 g fatty acid	[17]
Sunflower seed (11.2%)	400 (percentage increase)	[23]
Pasture	8.12 mg/100 g cheese	[38]
Pasture, 100 g/kg of sunflower oil/d	1.93 g/100 g fatty acid	[41]
Grass-fed animals	64·19 mg/100 g cheese	[74]
Fish oil (0.75% of dry matter)	2.41 g/100 g fatty acid	[75]
Natural spring pasture	0.76 g/100 g fatty acid	[78]
Pasture grazing	1.45 g/100 g fatty acid	[79]

CLA represents two major CLA isomers of C18:2 cis-9, trans-11 and trans-10, cis-12 isomer, TMR: total mixed ration, DM: dry matter, FA: fatty acid.

Table 3. Effect of feed modification on CLA content in milk's cheese.

with unknown geometric position. However, the two major peaks in that commercial CLA mixture were assumed the isomers c9, t11 and t10, c12. Later on, further research advances turned out to achieve the possible isomerization with specific isomers ratios [82]. Propylene glycol isomerization was another method to produce CLA from monounsaturated and poly-unsaturated oil fatty acids. The propylene glycol was used with KOH as a catalyst instead of ethylene alcohol for consumer safety reasons. Later, hexane was also used instead of ethylene/propylene glycol to facilitate the purification of required CLA isomers. Thus, the mixture of CLA isomers was marketed as free acids instead of n-3 concentrates [83]. Isomerization of mono-alkyl ester is a relatively recent effective quantitative method to produce CLA isomers by isomerizing methyl and ethyl esters of linolenic acids in presence of very small quantity of catalyst and virtually no solvent. Besides, thermal sigma tropic rearrangement by preceding the reaction below 100°C results in CLA isomer production.

1.6.2. Microbial CLA

Regarding the potential health effects, safe isomers selective processes are investigated for CLA production. Among these, bioprocess by microbial use is the potential method for production of CLA. Initially, the bacteria were divided into group A and group B depending on the type of reactions and the products as result of biohydrogenation. The bacteria of group A were able to hydrogenate linolenic acid and α-linolenic acid end product t11- C18:1. The group B bacteria were able to convert t11-C18:1 to end product stearic acid [84]. Besides ruminant bacteria, some bacterial strains from human/animal intestinal membrane, dairy products origins were isolated for CLA production. *Lactobacillus reuteri, Lactobacillus plantarum, Lactobacillus lrhamnosus, Lactobacillus brevis, Lactococcus lactis, Lactobacillus acidophilus, Propionibaterium freudenrehichii, Bifidobacterium, Streptococcus,* are capable for CLA production. Potential CLA producing strains such as bifidobacteria *Bifidobacterium,* lactobacilli, and pediococci have been selective for CLA production. The increasing interest in bifidobacteria as the natural inhabitant and useful in conversion of CLA fatty acid has been derived the attention of microbiologists [70]. Coakley et al. reported for the first time that the strains collection of bifidobacteria, lactobacilli, and pediococci were capable to convert LA into CLA isomers [41]. They sorted out the nine strains of bifidobacteria, which convert c9, t11 CLA from MRS culture supplemented with linoleic acids. Among these nine strains, *Bifidobacterium breve* is strong bio convertor of LA to 66% to c9, t11 CLA and 6.2% to t9, t11 CLA in only the culture supernatant [41, 85, 86]. Several studies have also reported the pivotal role of lactic acid bacteria in production of CLA from LA when grown on MRS, skim milk and cheddar cheese [75, 87, 88]. These bacteria have enzymatic conversion of LA to CLA by linoleate isomerase in their cell wall. *Lactobacillus reuteri* PYR8, *Clostridium sporogenes* and *Propionibacterium acnes* were reported to have putative polyunsaturated fatty acid PUFA linoleate isomerase function [89–91]. Several efforts were made to produce the CLA using *E. coli*, but none was capable to produce CLA. However, *Lactobacillus plantarum* AKU 1009a were found to produce t11-CLA, t10, c12-CLA and t9, t11-CLA with less known enzymatic action [85, 92, 93]. Later, the genetic mutation in linoleate isomerase enzyme machinery of strain plantrum AKU 1009a led to develop *E. coli* as catalysts to produce significant t9, t11-CLA with c9, t11-CLA [92, 94].

2. Bioavailability and clinical manifestation of enhanced CLA

The general availability of CLA from food sources has been summarized in **Table 4**. Recently, the manipulation of fatty acid profile of milk, meat, cheese and butter has been shown to confer beneficial impacts on human health. There are very few experimental studies that indicate the kinetic behavior of dietary CLA from naturally enhanced diary and meat products. The studies on kinetic behavior of polyunsaturated fatty acids (PUFAs) showed that the bioavailability and disposition of PUFA could be altered in some biologic fluids after the intake of enriched PUFA-rich food products. For example, previous studies with high-fat diet and low-fat diet containing 1% rumenic acid show higher and lower bioavailability of CLA content respectively which in return was more bioactive in reducing hyperinsulinemia [95]. The experimental rats group fed on CLA enriched butter had sixfold higher CLA content in liver compared to that of the control group, without having difference in dietary intake. The naturally enriched CLA butter consumption leads to increase the c9, t11-CLA serum concentrations and will as other PUFA without influencing the cholesterol content and blood TG [96, 97]. de Almeida et al. showed that the animals with synthetic CLA supplement diet have lower level of hyperinsulinemia, hyperglycemia and inflammatory proteins in retroperitoneal adipose tissue with high level of plasma HDL cholesterol [95]. While, other studies in which synthetic CLA mixture was used, report unhealthy effect of synthetic CLA as compared to that of naturally enriched CLA products, several authors have reported that using synthetic CLA in animal developed insulin resistance, hyperinsulinemia [97–98]. Thus, it is important to differentiate the bioavailability of CLA from different production sources, which ultimately determine the bio-functionalities of CLA from the health point of view. As commercial commercially produced CLA has predominant with mixture of 10-, 9,11-, 10,12-, and 11,13-isomers while natural CLA has 80–90% of 9,11-isomer. This difference in isomers composition is a major determinant of biological activities of CLA in diet and thus source. Furthermore,

Food Product	Fat (g)/serving	CLA(mg)/g fat	CLA (mg)/serving
Milk and milk products			
250 mL of milk (2% fat)	5.1	4.1	20.9
125 mL of condensed milk	14.1	7.0	98.7
250 mL of fermented buttermilk (2%)	5.2	5.4	28.1
175 g of plain yogurt (2–4% fat)	4.9	4.8	23.5
175 g of yogurt (1–2% fat)	2.7	4.4	11.9
50 g of processed cheese	12.3	5.0	61.5
50 g of cheddar cheese	16.6	4.1	68.1
15 mL of butter	11.7	4.7	55.0
125 mL cream	17.1	4.6	78.7
125 mL ice cream	11.8	3.6	42.5
Meat and meat products			
90 g of lamb meat	12.7	5.8	73.7
90 g of ground beef	12.3	4.3	52.9
90 g of veal	6.1	2.7	16.5
90 g of fresh ground turkey	6.5	2.6	16.9
90 g of chicken	12.1	0.9	10.9
90 g of pork	13.8	0.6	8.3
Large egg yolk	5.3	0.6	3.2
90 g of salmon	5.7	0.3	1.7
Vegetable oils			
15 mL of safflower oil	13.8	0.7	9.7
15 mL of sunflower oil	13.8	0.4	5.5

Table 4. Availability of CLA content from food products.

the bioavailability of CLA is measured either the total contents of CLA in blood circulation after ingestion or the total contents of CLA disposition in the liver, mammary fat, peritoneal fat and plasma. The composition of CLA isomers mixture can also influence the incorporation and bioavailability of CLA to tissue and organs. To date, most of the human studies evaluated by only blood measurements, which are different from animal models regarding the bioavailability and distribution modes of CLA according organs, model of dietary supplementation or enrichment [97, 99].

A very recent study by Rodriguez-Alcala et al. (2015) was conducted on oral absorption and disposition of CLA isomers from naturally enriched goat milk cheese conducted to evaluate the bioavailability of CLA. The oral doses of 153 mg vaccenic acid, 46 mg rumenic acid were fed to rats on kilogram body weight basis. The maximum concentration value of vaccenic acid and rumenic acid were 18.76 and 63.42 µg/mL in plasma and 7.60 and 26.66 µg/g in erythrocytes, respectively, suggesting that CLA-enriched dairy fat produced by dietary manipulation may be well absorbed for better health effects in humans as compared to synthetic CLA [9]. It was observed that the rats fed on butter selectively absorbed more CLA. The accumulation was fourfold more higher for total CLA in mammary gland and tissues compared to rats fed on synthetic free fatty acids while taking the same dietary intake [100]. The studies on transfer efficiency of a CLA showed that bioavailability of the 9, 11-CLA isomer was twofold more as compared to 10, 12-CLA isomer [97]. While feeding of commercial CLA to pigs showed that c9, t11-isomer preferentially incorporate to liver and c11, t13-isomer into heart. Another study showed that the serum bioavailability of synthetic CLA was low when was inducted to pig feed for 15 days dietary treatments. The results were in increase of 10–30-fold mono-CLA isomers (c9, t11-c15-18:3 + c9-t13-c15-18:3) in the heart, kidneys and liver indicating the trend of incorporation of conjugated CLA isomers, which depends on the structure and source of the conjugated fatty acids [47]. The rats fed during the mammary gland development period show that naturally enriched CLA was more potent in reducing 22% epithelial mass, 30% terminal end bud density, 30% proliferation and 53% tumor yield of mammary glands. The consumers have the options for choosing CLA to increase CLA intake from synthetic CLA pill or produced by diet modification in dairy and meat products. The relative health value benefits of CLA from ruminant, microbes, and synthetic sources are uncertain regarding the bioavailability and functional disposition in human [100, 101].

3. Conclusion

Enhanced or enriched dairy fats produced by dietary manipulation are considered well-absorbed and bioactive source of essential fatty acids with beneficial health effects in humans. However, most of the studies related to effect of CLA on human health were conducted on commercial CLA that was differentially available and dispersed in body organs and tissues and hence have different health effects. Further, there are not conclusive studies on the moderation of CLA and its dietary source on average human intake. The extrapolation from rat animal models to human intake must be taken with cautions due to difference in dietary requirements. To meet recommended intake of CLA, several efforts have been made to enhance the level of CLA naturally and natural enhanced CLA in dairy food is more health effective. The manipulation of dairy ration type and composition seems to be one of the most suitable strategies for enhancement of CLA in enriched dairy products. Manipulation of the animal's diet can result in up to 8- to 10-fold increase in the concentration of CLA in milk. As consumers become more conscious of the link between diet and health, milk designed to have enhanced levels of CLA may provide new market opportunities for milk and milk products such as butter and cheese.

Acknowledgements

We would like to acknowledge that Government College University Faisalabad and its IT department provided us kind permission to use digital library and access to research data.

Conflict of interest

All authors declare no conflict of interest for any purpose.

Author details

Nazir Ahmad[1]*, Muhammad Kamran Khan[1], Muhammad Imran[1],
Muhammad Nadeem Suleman[2] and Sufyan Afzal[1]

*Address all correspondence to: drnazirahmad@gcuf.edu.pk

1 Institute of Home and Food Sciences, Faculty of Science and Technology, Government
College University, Faisalabad, Pakistan

2 Advanced Animal Nutrition, Punjab Small Industrial Corporation, Faisalabad, Pakistan

References

[1] Chin SF, Liu W, Storkson JM, Ha YL, Pariza MW. Dietary sources of conjugated dienoic
isomers of linoleic acid, a newly recognized class of anticarcinogens. Journal of Food
Composition and Analysis. 1992;**5**:185-197. DOI: 10.1016/08891575(92)90037

[2] Pariza MW, Park Y, Cook ME. The biologically active isomers of conjugated linoleic acid.
Progress in Lipid Research. 2017;**40**:283-298. DOI: 10.1016/S0163-7827(01)00008

[3] Fritsche J, Rickert R, Steinhart H. Conjugated linoleic acid (CLA) isomers: Formation,
analysis, amounts in foods, and dietary intake. In: Christie WW, Sebedio JL, Adlo R, editors. Advances in Conjugated Linoleic Acid Research. 2nd ed. CRC Press; 1999. pp. 378-
396. DOI: 10.1002/(SICI)1521-4133(199908)101:8

[4] Fritsche J, Fritsche S, Solomon MB, Mossoba MM, Yurawecz MP, Morehouse K, Ku
Y. Quantitative determination of conjugated linoleic acid isomers in beef fat. European
Journal of Lipid Science and Technology. 2000;**102**:667-672. DOI: 10.1002/1438-9312
(200011)102:11

[5] Mir PS, McAllister TA, Scott S, Aalhus J, Baron V, McCartney D, Charmley E, Goonewardene
L, Basarab J, Okine E, Weselake RJ, Mir Z. Conjugated linoleic acid-enriched beef production. The American Journal of Clinical Nutrition. 2004;**79**:1207-1211. DOI: 10.1093/
ajcn/79.6.1207S

[6] Zlatanos SN, Laskaridis K, Sagredos A. Conjugated linoleic acid content of human
plasma. Lipids in Health and Disease. 2008;**7**:34. DOI: 10.1186/1476-511X-7-34

[7] Elgersma A, Tamminga S, Ellen G. Modifying milk composition through forage. Animal
Feed Science and Technology. 2006;**131**:207-225. DOI: 10.1016/j.anifeedsci.2006.06.012

[8] Ponnampalam EN, Butler KL, Jacob RH, Pethick DW, Ball AJ, Edwards JE, Geesink G,
Hopkins DL. Health beneficial long chain omega-3 fatty acid levels in Australian lamb

managed under extensive finishing systems. Meat Science. 2014;**96**:1104-1110. DOI: 10.1016/j.meatsci.2013.04.007

[9] Rodriguez-Alcala LM, Ares I, Fontecha J, Juarez M, Castellano V, Martinez Larranaga MR, Anadon A, Martinez MA. Oral absorption and disposition of alpha-linolenic, rumenic and vaccenic acids after administration as a naturally enriched goat dairy fat to rats. Lipids. 2015;**50**:659-666. DOI: 10.1007/s11745-015-4034-8

[10] Kepler CR, Hirons KP, McNeill JJ, Tove SB. Intermediates and products of the biohydrogenation of linoleic acid by Butyrinvibrio fibrisolvens. The Journal of Biological Chemistry. 1996;**241**:1350-1354

[11] Parodi PW. Conjugated linoleic acid and other anticarcinogenic agents of bovine milk fat. Journal of Dairy Science. 1999;**82**:1339-1349. DOI: 10.3168/jds.S0022-0302(99)75358-0

[12] Griinari JM, Corl BA, Lacy SH, Chouinard PY, Nurmela KV, Bauman DE. Conjugated linoleic acid is synthesized endogenously in lactating dairy cows by Delta (9)-desaturase. The Journal of Nutrition. 2000;**130**:2285-2291. DOI: 10.1093/jn/130.9.2285

[13] Santora JE, Palmquist DL, Roehrig KL. Trans-vaccenic acid is desaturated to conjugated linoleic acid in mice. The Journal of Nutrition. 2000;**130**:208-215. DOI: 10.1093/jn/130.2.208

[14] Dhiman TR, Satter LD, Pariza MW, Galli MP, Albright K, Tolosa MX. Conjugated linoleic acid (CLA) content of milk from cows offered diets rich in linoleic and linolenic acid. Journal of Dairy Science. 2000;**83**:1016-1027. DOI: 10.3168/jds. S0022-0302(00)74966-6

[15] Bauman DE, Griinari JM. Nutritional regulation of milk fat synthesis. Annual Review of Nutrition. 2003;**23**:203-227. DOI: 10.1146/annurev.nutr.23.011702.073408

[16] Khanal RC, Olson KC. Factors affecting conjugated linoleic acid (CLA) content in milk, meat, and egg: A review. PJN. 2004;**3**:82-98. DOI: 10.3923/pjn.2004.82.98

[17] Khanal RC, Dhiman TR, Ure AL, Brennand CP, Boman RL, McMahon DJ. Consumer acceptability of conjugated linoleic acid-enriched milk and cheddar cheese from cows grazing on pasture. Journal of Dairy Science. 2005;**88**:1837-1847. DOI: 10.3168/jds.S0022-0302(05)72858-7

[18] Moon HS, Lee HG, Chung CS, Choi YJ, Cho CS. Physico-chemical modifications of conjugated linoleic acid for ruminal protection and oxidative stability. Nutrition and Metabolism. 2008;**5**:16. DOI: 10.1186/1743-7075-5-16

[19] Bouattour MA, Casals R, Albanell E, Such X, Caja G. Feeding soybean oil to dairy goats increases conjugated linoleic acid in milk. Journal of Dairy Science. 2008;**91**:2399-2407. DOI: 10.3168/jds.2007-0753

[20] Martinez Marin AL, Gomez Cortes P, Gomez Castro AG, Juarez M, Perez Alba LM, Perez Hernandez M, De La Fuente MA. Animal performance and milk fatty acid profile of dairy goats fed diets with different unsaturated plant oils. Journal of Dairy Science. 2011;**94**:5359-5368. DOI: 10.3168/jds.2011-4569

[21] Nudda A, Battacone G, Boaventura NO, Cannas A, Francesconi AHD, Atzori AS, Pulina G. Feeding strategies to design the fatty acid profile of sheep milk and cheese. Revista Brasileira de Zootecnia. 2014;**43**:445-456. DOI: 10.1590/S1516-35982014000800008

[22] Loor JJ, Ferlay A, Ollier A, Doreau M, Chilliard Y. Relationship among trans and conjugated fatty acids and bovine milk fat yield due to dietary concentrate and linseed oil.
Journal of Dairy Science. 2005;**88**:726-740. DOI: 10.3168/jds.S0022-0302(05)72736-3

[23] Cruz-Hernandez C, Kramer JK, Kennelly JJ, Glimm DR, Sorensen BM, Okine EK, Goonewardene LA, Weselake RJ. Evaluating the conjugated linoleic acid and trans 18:1 isomer in milk fat of dairy cows fed increasing amounts of sunflower oil and a constant
level of fish oil. Journal of Dairy Science. 2007;**90**:3786-3801. DOI: 10.3168/jds.2006-698

[24] Abbeddou SR, Richter B, Hess EK, Kreuzer HD. Modification of milk fatty acid composition by feeding forages and agro-industrial byproducts from dry areas to Awassi sheep.
Journal of Dairy Science. 2011;**94**:4657-4668. DOI: 10.3168/jds.2011-4154

[25] Bell JA, Griinari JM, Kennelly JJ. Effect of safflower oil, flaxseed oil, monensin, and vitamin E on concentration of conjugated linoleic acid in bovine milk fat. Journal of Dairy
Science. 2006;**89**:733-748. DOI: 10.3168/jds.S0022-0302(06)72135-X

[26] Morales R, Ungerfeld EM. Use of tannins to improve fatty acids profile of meat and milk
quality in ruminants: A review. Chilean Journal of Agricultural Research. 2015;**75**:239-
248. DOI: 10.4067/S0718-58392015000200014

[27] Tyagi AKK, Dhiman N, Kaur TR, Singhal H, Kanwajia SKKK. Enhancement of the
conjugated linoleic acid content of buffalo milk and milk products through green fodder feeding. Animal Feed Science and Technology. 2007;**133**:351-358. DOI: 10.1016/j.
anifeedsci.2006.05.003

[28] Zened A, Enjalbert F, Nicot MC, Meynadier AT. In vitro study of dietary factors affecting
the biohydrogenation shift from trans-11 to trans-10 fatty acids in the rumen of dairy
cows. International Journal of Research in BioSciences. 2012;**6**:459-467. DOI: 10.1017/
S1751731111001777

[29] Zened A, Meynadier AT, Najar T, Enjalbert F. Effects of oil and natural or synthetic
vitamin E on ruminal and milk fatty acid profiles in cows receiving a high-starch diet.
Journal of Dairy Science. 2012;**95**:5916-5926. DOI: 10.3168/jds.2012-5326

[30] Toral PGC, Rouel Y, Leskinen J, Shingfield H, Bernard LKJ. Comparison of the nutritional regulation of milk fat secretion and composition in cows and goats. Journal of
Dairy Science. 2015;**98**:7277-7297. DOI: 10.3168/jds.2015-9649

[31] Bodkowski R, Czyż K, Kupczyński B, Patkowska-Sokoła R, Nowakowski P, Wiliczkiewicz
A. Lipid complex effect on fatty acid profile and chemical composition of cow milk and
cheese. Journal of Dairy Science. 2016;**99**:57-67. DOI: 10.3168/jds.2015-9321

[32] Kholif SM, El-Shewy AA, Morsy TA, Abd El-Rahman HH. Variations in protein and fat
contents and their fractions in milk from two species fed different forages. Journal of
Animal Physiology and Animal Nutrition. 2015;**99**:79-84. DOI: 10.1111/jpn.12214

[33] Pirondini M, Colombini S, Mele M, Malagutti L, Rapetti L, Galassi G, Crovetto GM.
Effect of dietary starch concentration and fish oil supplementation on milk yield and
composition, diet digestibility, and methane emissions in lactating dairy cows. Journal
of Dairy Science. 2015;**98**:357-372. DOI: 10.3168/jds.2014-8092

[34] Suksombat W, Thanh LP, Meeprom C, Mirattanaphrai R. Effects of linseed oil or whole linseed supplementation on performance and milk fatty acid composition of lactating dairy cows. Asian-Australasian Journal of Animal Sciences. 2014;**27**:951-959. DOI: 10.5713/ajas.2013.13665

[35] Paradis C, Berthiaume R, Lafreniere C, Gervais R, Chouinard PY. Conjugated linoleic acid content in adipose tissue of calves suckling beef cows on pasture and supplemented with raw or extruded soybeans. Journal of Animal Science. 2008;**86**:1624-1636. DOI: 10.2527/jas.2007-0702

[36] Vafa TS, Naserian AA, Heravi MAR, Valizadeh R, Mesgaran MD. Effect of supplementation of fish and canola oil in the diet on milk fatty acid composition in early lactating Holstein cows. Asian-Australasian Journal of Animal Sciences. 2012;**25**:311-319. DOI: 10.5713/ajas.2010.10014

[37] Castro T, Manso T, Jimeno V, Del AM, Mantecón AR. Effects of dietary sources of vegetable fats on performance of dairy ewes and conjugated linoleic acid (CLA) in milk. Small Ruminant Research. 2009;**84**:47-53. DOI: 10.1016/j.smallrumres.2009.05.005

[38] Kim JH, Kwon OJ, Choi NJ, Oh SJ, Jeong HY, Song MK, Jeong I, Kim YJ. Variations in conjugated linoleic acid (CLA) content of processed cheese by lactation time, feeding regimen, and ripening. Journal of Agricultural and Food Chemistry. 2009;**57**:3235-3239. DOI: 10.1021/jf803838

[39] Murphy JJ, Coakley M, Stanton C. Supplementation of dairy cows with a fish oil containing supplement and sunflower oil to increase the CLA content of milk produced at pasture. Livestock Science. 2008;**116**:332-337. DOI: doi.org/10.1016/j.livsci.2008.02.003

[40] AbuGhazaleh AA. Effect of fish oil and sunflower oil supplementation on milk conjugated linoleic acid content for grazing dairy cows. Animal Feed Science and Technology. 2008;**141**:220-232. DOI: 10.1016/j.anifeedsci.2007.06.027

[41] Coakley M, Barrett E, Murphy JJ, Ross RP, Devery R, Stanton C. Cheese manufacture with milk with elevated conjugated linoleic acid levels caused by dietary manipulation. Journal of Dairy Science. 2007;**90**:2919-2927. DOI: 10.3168/jds.2006-584

[42] Shingfield KJ, Reynolds CK, Hervas G, Griinari JM, Grandison AS, Beever DE. Examination of the persistency of milk fatty acid composition responses to fish oil and sunflower oil in the diet of dairy cows. Journal of Dairy Science. 2006;**89**:714-732. DOI: 10.3168/jds.S0022-0302(06)72134-8

[43] Ward AT, Wittenberg KM, Froebe HM, Przybylski R, Malcolmson L. Fresh forage and Solin supplementation on conjugated linoleic acid levels in plasma and milk. Journal of Dairy Science. 2003;**86**:1742-1750. DOI: 10.3168/jds.S0022-0302(03)73760-6

[44] Abu-Ghazaleh AA, Schingoethe DJ, Hippen AR, Whitlock LA. Feeding fish meal and extruded soybeans enhances the conjugated linoleic acid (CLA) content of Milk1. Journal of Dairy Science. 2002;**85**:624-631. DOI: 10.3168/jds.S0022-0302(02)74116-7

[45] Chilliard Y, Glasser F, Ferlay A, Bernard L, Rouel J, Doreau M. Diet, rumen biohydrogenation and nutritional quality of cow and goat milk fat. European Journal of Lipid Science and Technology. 2007;**09**(8):828-855. DOI: 10.1002/ejlt.200700080

[46] Kelly ML, Berry JR, Dwyer DA, Griinari JM, Chouinard PY, Van AME, Bauman DE. Dietary fatty acid sources affect conjugated linoleic acid concentrations in milk from lactating dairy cows. The Journal of Nutrition. 1998;**128**:881-885. DOI: 10.1093/jn/128.5.881

[47] Chouinard PY, Corneau L, Barbano DM, Metzger LE, Bauman DE. Conjugated linoleic acids alter milk fatty acid composition and inhibit milk fat secretion in dairy cows. The Journal of Nutrition. 1999;**129**:1579-1584. DOI: 10.1093/jn/129.8.1579

[48] Pereira ACSC, Santos MVD, Aferri G, Corte RRPDS, Silva SDLE, Júnior JEDF, Leme PR, Rennó FP. Lipid and selenium sources on fatty acid composition of intramuscular fat and muscle selenium concentration of Nellore steers. Revista Brasileira de Zootecnia. 2012;**41**(11):2357-2363. DOI: 10.1590/S1516-35982012001100009

[49] Mapiye C, Turner TD, Basarab JA, Baron VS, Aalhus JL, Dugan MER. Subcutaneous fatty acid composition of steers finished as weanlings or yearlings with and without growth promotants. Journal of Animal Science and Biotechnology. 2013;**4**:41-41. DOI: 10.1186/2049-1891-4-41

[50] Adrián CRM, Rojas C, Cancino D. Beef production from dairy bulls under two different production systems and its effect on the fatty acid profile and beef quality. Chilean Journal of Agricultural Research. 2014;**74**(3). DOI: 10.4067/S0718-58392014000300017

[51] Ladeira MM, Santarosa LC, Chizzotti ML, Ramos EM, Neto ORM, Oliveira DM, Carvalho JRR, Lopes LS, Ribeiro JS. Fatty acid profile, color and lipid oxidation of meat from young bulls fed ground soybean or rumen protected fat with or without monensin. Meat Science. 2014;**96**:597-560. DOI: 10.1016/j.meatsci.2013.04.062

[52] Joele P, Lourenço LFH, Ribeiro ASC, Meller LH. Buffalo meat from animals fed with agro industrial in Eastern Amazon. Archivos de Zootecnia. 2014;**63**(242):359-369. DOI: 10.4321/S0004-05922014000200014

[53] Fiorentini G, Lage JF, Carvalho IPC, Messana JD, Canesin RC, Reis RA, Berchielli TT. Lipid sources with different fatty acid profile alters the fatty acid profile and quality of beef from confined Nellore steers. Asian-Australasian Journal of Animal Sciences. 2015;**28**(7):976-986. DOI: 10.5713/ajas.14.0893

[54] Gómez I, Beriain MJ, Mendizabal JA, Realini C, Purroy A. Shelf life of ground beef enriched with omega-3 and/or conjugated linoleic acid and use of grape seed extract to inhibit lipid oxidation. Food Science & Nutrition. 2015;**4**:67-79. DOI: 10.1002/fsn3.251

[55] De La Torre A, Gruffat D, Durand D, Micol D, Peyron A, Scislowski V, Bauchart D. Factors influencing proportion and composition of CLA in beef. Meat Science. 2006;**73**:258-268. DOI: 10.1016/j.meatsci.2005.11.025

[56] Enser M, Scollan ND, Choi NJ, Kurt E, Hallet K, Wood JD. Effect of dietary lipid on the content of conjugated linoleic acid (CLA) in beef muscle. Journal of Animal Science. 1999;**69**:143-146. DOI: 10.1017/S1357729800051171

[57] Jambrenghi MAC, Giannico F, Cappiello G, Vonghia G. Effect of goat production systems on meat quality and conjugated linoleic acid (CLA) content in suckling kids. Italian Journal of Animal Science. 2007;**6**:612-614. DOI: 10.4081/ijas.2007.1s.612

[58] Karabacak A, Aytekin I, Boztepe S. Fatty acid composition and conjugated linoleic acid content in different carcass parts of Akkaraman lambs. The Scientific World Journal. 2015;**2014**:1-5. DOI: 10.1155/2014/821904

[59] Gonzalez F, Muiño R, Pereira V, Martinez D, Castillo C, Hernández J, Benedito JL. Milk yield and reproductive performance of dairy heifers and cows supplemented with polyunsaturated fatty acids. Pesquisa Agropecuária Brasileira. 2015;**50**:306-312. DOI: 10.1590/S0100-204X2015000400006

[60] Angulo J, Mahecha L, Nuernberg K, Nuernberg G, Dannenberger D, Olivera M, Boutinaud M, Leroux C, Albrecht E, Bernard L. Effects of polyunsaturated fatty acids from plant oils and algae on milk fat yield and composition are associated with mammary lipogenic and SREBF1 gene expression. International Journal of Research in BioSciences. 2012;**6**:1961-1972. DOI: 10.1017/S1751731112000845

[61] Steen RWJ, Porter MG. The effects of high-concentrate diets and pasture on the concentration of conjugated linoleic acid in beef muscle and subcutaneous fat. Grass and Forage Science. 2003;**58**:50-57. DOI: 10.1046/j.1365-2494.2003.00351

[62] Scollan N, Hocquette JF, Nuernberg K, Dannenberger D, Richardson I, Moloney A. Innovations in beef production systems that enhance the nutritional and health value of beef lipids and their relationship with meat quality. Meat Science. 2006;**74**:17-33. DOI: 10.1016/j.meatsci.2006.05.002

[63] Griswold KE, Apgar GA, Robinson RA, Jacobson BN, Johnson D, Woody HD. Effectiveness of short-term feeding strategies for altering conjugated linoleic acid content of beef. Journal of Animal Science. 2003;**81**:1862-1871. DOI: 10.2527/2003.8171862x

[64] Mir PS, Mir Z, Kuber PS, Gaskins CT, Martin EL, Dodson MV, Elias Calles JA, Johnson KA, Busboom JR, Wood AJ, Pittenger GJ, Reeves JJ. Growth, carcass characteristics, muscle conjugated linoleic acid (CLA) content, and response to intravenous glucose challenge in high percentage Wagyu, Wagyu×Limousin, and Limousin steers fed sunflower oil-containing diets. Journal of Animal Science. 2002;**80**:29996-23004. DOI: 10.2527/ 2002.80112996x

[65] Beaulieu AD, Drackley JK, Merchen NR. Concentrations of conjugated linoleic acid (cis-9, trans-11-octadecadienoic acid) are not increased in tissue lipids of cattle fed a high-concentrate diet supplemented with soybean oil. Journal of Animal Science. 2002; **80**:847-861. DOI: 10.2527/2002.803847x

[66] Madron MS, Peterson DG, Dwyer DA, Corl BA, Baumgard LH, Beermann DH, Bauman DE. Effect of extruded full-fat soybeans on conjugated linoleic acid content of intramuscular, intermuscular, and subcutaneous fat in beef steers. Journal of Animal Science. 2002;**80**:1135-1143. DOI: 10.2527/2002.8041135x

[67] Poulson CS, Dhiman TR, Cornforth D, Olson KC. Conjugated linoleic acid content of beef from cattle fed diets containing high grain, CLA, or raised on forages. Livestock Production Science. 2001;**52**:87-90. DOI: 10.1016/j.livprodsci.2004.07.012

[68] French P, Stanton C, Lawless F, O'Riordan EG, Monahan FJ, Caffrey PJ, Moloney AP. Fatty acid composition, including conjugated linoleic acid, of intramuscular fat from

steers offered grazed grass, grass silage, or concentrate-based diets. Journal of Animal Science. 2000;78:2849-2855

[69] Mir PS, Mir Z, Kuber PS, Gaskins CT, Martin EL, Dodson MV, Elias Calles JA, Johnson KA, Busboom JR, Wood AJ, Pittenger GP, Reeves JJ. Growth, carcass characteristics, muscle linoleic acid (CLA) content, and response to intravenous glucose challenge in high percentage Wagyu, WagyuX limousine, and Limousin steers fed sunflower oil-containing diets. Journal of Animal Science. 2002b;80:2996-3004

[70] Gómez-Cortés P, Bach A, Luna P, Juárez M, de la Fuente MA. Effects of extruded linseed supplementation on n-3 fatty acids and conjugated linoleic acid in milk and cheese from ewes. Journal of Dairy Science. 2009;92:4122-4134. DOI: 10.3168/jds.2008-1909

[71] Bodas R, Manso T, Mantecón ÁR, Juárez M, De la Fuente MÁ, Gómez-Cortés P. Comparison of the fatty acid profiles in cheeses from ewes fed diets supplemented with different plant oils. Journal of Agricultural and Food Chemistry. 2010;58:10493-10502. DOI: 10.1021/jf101760u

[72] Pintus S, Carta EMG, Cordeddu L, Batetta B, Accossu S, Pistis D, Uda S, Ghiani ME, Secchiari P, Almerighi G, Pintus P, Mele M, Banni S. Sheep cheese naturally enriched in a-linolenic, conjugated linoleic and vaccenic acids improves the lipid profile and reduces anandamide in the plasma of hypercholesterolaemic subjects. British Journal of Nutrition. 2013;109:1453-1462. DOI: 10.1017/S0007114512003224

[73] Allred SL, Dhiman TR, Brennand CP, Khanal RC, McMahon DJ, Luchini ND. Milk and cheese from cows fed calcium salts of palm and fish oil alone or in combination with soybean products. Journal of Dairy Science. 2006;89:234-248. DOI: 10.3168/jds.S0022-0302(06)72088-4

[74] McAfee AJ, McSorley EM, Cuskelly GJ, Fearon AM, Moss BW, Beattie JAM, Wallace JMW, Bonham MP, Strain JJ. Red meat from animals offered a grass diet increases plasma and platelet n-3 PUFA in healthy consumers. British Journal of Nutrition. 2011;105:80-89. DOI: 10.1017/S0007114510003090

[75] Mohan MS, Anand S, Kalscheur KF, Hassan AN, Hippen AR. Starter cultures and cattle feed manipulation enhance conjugated linoleic acid concentrations in cheddar cheese. Journal of Dairy Science. 2013;96:2081-2094. DOI: 10.3168/jds.2012-6101

[76] dos Santosa KM, Bomfima MA, Vieira AD, Benevidesa SD, Saad SM, Buritia FC, Egito AS. Probiotic caprine Coalho cheese naturally enriched in conjugated linoleic acid as a vehicle for *Lactobacillus acidophilus* and beneficial fatty acids. International Dairy Journal. 2011;24:107-112. DOI: 10.1016/j.idairyj.2011.12.001

[77] Medeiros E, Queiroga R, Oliveira M, Medeiros A, Sabedot M, Bomfim M, Madruga M. Fatty acid profile of cheese from dairy goats fed a diet enriched with castor, sesame and faveleira vegetable oils. Molecules. 2014;19:992-1003. DOI: 10.3390/molecules19010992

[78] Van Nieuwenhove CP, Oliszewski R, González SN. Fatty acid composition and conjugated linoleic acid content of cow and goat cheeses from Northwest Argentina. Journal of Food Quality. 2009;32:303-314. DOI: 10.1111/j.1745-4557.2009.00258.x

[79] Tornambé G, Cornu A, Pradel P, Kondjoyan N, Carnat AP, Petit M, Martin B. Changes in terpene content in milk from pasture-fed cows. Journal of Dairy Science. 2006;**89**:2309-2319. DOI: 10.3168/jds.S0022-0302(06)72302-5

[80] Burr OG, U.S.Patent 2, 242, 230; 1941

[81] Bradley TF, U.S. Patent, 2, 350, 358; 1944

[82] Christie WW, Dobson G, Gunstone FD. Isomers in commercial samples of conjugated linoleic acid. Lipids. 1997;**32**:1231. DOI: 10.1007/s11745-997-0158-1

[83] Yurawecz MP, Sehat N, Mossoba MM, Roach JA, Kramer JK, Ku Y. Variations in isomer distribution in commercially available conjugated linoleic acid. Lipids. 1999;**101**:277-282. DOI: 10.1002/(SICI)1521-4133(199908)101:8

[84] Kemp P, Lander DJ. Hydrogenation in vitro of alpha linolenic acid to stearic acid by mixed cultures of pure strains of rumen bacteria. Journal of General Microbiology. 1984;**130**:527-533. DOI: 10.1099/00221287-130-3-527

[85] Rosberg-Cody E, Ross R, Hussey S, Ryan C, Murphy B, Fitzgerald GF, Devery R, Stanton C. Mining the microbiota of the neonatal gastrointestinal tract for conjugated linoleic acid-producing bifidobacteria. Applied and Environmental Microbiology. 2004;**70**:4635-4641. DOI: 10.1128/AEM.70.8.4635-4641.2004

[86] Gorissen L, Raes K, Weckx S, Dannenberger D, Leroy F, De Vuyst L, De Smet S. Production of conjugated linoleic acid and conjugated linolenic acid isomers by Bifidobacterium species. Applied Microbiology and Biotechnology. 2010;**87**:2257-2266. DOI: 10.1007/s00253-010-2713-1

[87] Alonso L, Cuesta E, Gilliland S. Production of free conjugated linoleic acid by *Lactobacillus acidophilus* and *Lactobacillus casei* of human intestinal origin. Journal of Dairy Science. 2003;**86**:1941-1946. DOI: 10.3168/jds.S0022-0302(03)73781-3

[88] Ye S, Yu T, Yang H, Li L, Wang H, Xiao S, Wang J. Optimal culture conditions for producing conjugated linoleic acid in skim-milk by co-culture of different *Lactobacillus strains*. Annales de Microbiologie. 2013;**63**:707-717. DOI: 10.1007/s13213-012-0523-7

[89] Rosson RA, Grund AD, Deng MD, Sanchez-Riera F. Linoleateisomerase. Patent 6743609, United States, 2004

[90] Liavonchanka A, Hornung E, Feussner I, Rudolph MG. Structure and mechanism of the *Propionibacterium acnes* polyunsaturated fatty acid isomerase. Proceedings of the National Academy of Sciences of the United States of America. 2006;**103**:2576-2581. DOI: 10.1073/pnas.0510144103

[91] Peng SS, Deng MD, Grund AD, Rosson RA. Purification and characterization of a membrane-bound linoleic acid isomerase from *Clostridium sporogenes*. Enzyme and Microbial Technology. 2007;**40**:831-839. DOI: 10.1016/j.enzmictec.2006.06.020

[92] Kishino S, Ogawa J, Yokozeki K, Shimizu S. Linoleic acid isomerase in *Lactobacillus plantarum* AKU1009a proved to be a multi-component enzyme system requiring

oxidoreduction cofactors. Bioscience, Biotechnology, and Biochemistry. 2011;**75**:318-322. DOI: 10.1271/bbb.100699

[93] Kishino S, Takeuchi M, Park SB, Hirata A, Kitamura N, Kunisawa J, Kiyono H, Iwamoto R, Isobe Y, Arita M. Polyunsaturated fatty acid saturation by gut lactic acid bacteria affecting host lipid composition. Proceedings of the National Academy of Sciences. 2013;**110**:17808-17813. DOI: 10.1073/pnas.1312937110

[94] Volkov A, Khoshnevis S, Neumann P, Herrfurth C, Wohlwend D, Ficner R, Feussner I. Crystal structure analysis of a fatty acid double-bond hydratase from *Lactobacillus acidophilus*. Acta Crystallographica, Section D: Biological Crystallography. 2013;**69**:648-657. DOI: 10.1107/S0907444913000991

[95] De Almeida MM, Luquetti SCPD, Sabarense CM, Corrêa JODA, dos Reis LG, Da Conceição EPS, Lisboa PC, De Moura EG, Gameiro J, Da Gama MAS, Lopes FCF, Garcia RMG. Butter naturally enriched in cis-9, trans-11 CLA prevents hyperinsulinemia and increases both serum HDL cholesterol and triacylglycerol levels in rats. Lipids in Health and Disease. 2014;**13**:200. DOI: 10.1186/1476-511X-13-200

[96] Tricon S, Burdge GC, Jones EL, Russell JJ, El-Khazen S, Moretti E, Hall WL, Gerry AB, Leake DS, Grimble RF, Williams CM, Calder PC, Yaqoob P. Effects of dairy products naturally enriched with cis-9, trans-11 conjugated linoleic acid on the blood lipid profile in healthy middle-aged men. The American Journal of Clinical Nutrition. 2006;**83**:744-753. DOI: 10.1093/ajcn/83.4.744

[97] Haug A, Sjogren P, Holland N, Muller H, Kjos NP, Taugbol O, Fjerdingby N, Biong AS, Olsen SE, Harstad OM. Effects of butter naturally enriched with conjugated linoleic acid and vaccenic acid on blood lipids and LDL particle size in growing pigs. Lipids in Health and Disease. 2008;**7**:31. DOI: 10.1186/1476-511X-7-31

[98] Clément L, Poirier H, Niot I, Bocher V, Guerre-Millo M, Krief S, Staels B, Besnard P. Dietary trans-10, cis-12 conjugated linoleic acid induces hyperinsulinemia and fatty liver in the mouse. Journal of Lipid Research. 2002;**43**:1400-1409. DOI: 10.1194/jlr.M20008-JLR200

[99] Martins SV, Lopes PA, Alves SP, Alfaia CM, Castro MF, Bessa RJ, Prates JA. Dietary CLA combined with palm oil or ovine fat differentially influences fatty acid deposition in tissues of obese Zucker rats. Lipids. 2012;**47**:47-58. DOI: 10.1007/s11745-011-3626-1

[100] Cleland LG, Gibson RA, Pedler J, James MJ. Paradoxical effect of n-3-containing vegetable oils on long-chain n-3 fatty acids in rat heart. Lipids. 2005;**40**:995-998. DOI: 10.1007/s11745-005-1461-6

[101] Castellano CA, Plourde M, Briand SI, Angers P, Giguere A, Matte JJ. Safety of dietary conjugated alpha-linolenic acid (CLNA) in a neonatal pig model. Food and Chemical Toxicology. 2014;**64**:119-125. DOI: 10.1016/j.fct.2013.11.025

Emergence of Antimicrobial Resistance, Causes, Molecular Mechanisms, and Prevention Strategies: A Bovine Perspective

Muhammad Ashraf, Behar-E -Mustafa,
Shahid-Ur -Rehman, Muhammad Khalid Bashir and
Muhammad Adnan Ashraf

Additional information is available at the end of the chapter

http://dx.doi.org/10.5772/intechopen.79757

Abstract

Emergence of the resistance in microbial population is a major threat to both animal and human health. In bovine, the development of microbial resistance is a persistent threat for health especially in the form of zoonotic pandemics due to viral and multidrug bacterial resistance. Mechanisms of antimicrobial resistance in microbes are of natural as well as acquired origin. There are half dozen molecular mechanisms identified that possibly cause the emergence and transfer of antimicrobial resistance within and between different bacterial genera. These mechanisms include degradation of the antibacterial drug by the bacterial enzymes, reduced permeability of the drug by bacteria, increased efflux of the drug, modification of drug target and use of alternative pathways by bacterial cells. Various assays viz. disk diffusion test and E-test, focusing on minimum inhibitory concentration of antimicrobials, have been employed to detect the antimicrobial resistance in microbes. The most important factor responsible for the development of multidrug resistance in bovine pathogenic microbes is irrational use of the antibiotics. Antibiotics are necessary evil, so judicious use of antibiotics, early detection of infections, vaccination, use of immune-modulators and medicinal plants or their derivatives are some of the strategies to reduce the possible emergence of antimicrobial resistance.

Keywords: microbes, resistance, pandemic, zoonotic, antibiotic

1. Introduction

Antimicrobial compounds include antibiotics as well as many other substances which are used to kill or inhibit the growth (multiplication) of bacteria. But nowadays, many bacteria causing diseases of pandemic (e.g., tuberculosis) importance are increasingly developing the resistance against a myriad of the antimicrobial compounds which, in terms, is leading to the ineffective treatment of many fatal human and animal disease outbreaks.

1.1. Antimicrobial resistance in microbes

The idea of using antimicrobial compounds was originally proposed by Paul Ehrlich in 1908 who proposed to use some chemicals which he originally thought as "magic bullet" to kill the bacteria specifically with a minimum harm to the host (animals and humans). He used SilverSan to treat an infectious disease in humans transmitted through sexual contact known as syphilis. This was the first time that a chemical was used to treat the microbial infections. Since the discovery of the first antibiotic, penicillin (1920s), researcher worked diligently to find new antibiotics, and this leads to the discovery of many new antibiotics, e.g., tetracycline, gentamicin, and chloramphenicol. Antibiotics are compounds which are produced by one microbe, and they are used to kill the other microbial spp. So, till 1950 a majority of infectious diseases in humans were treatable by using these antibiotics [1].

However, unfortunately, soon after the clinical use of antibiotics, a phenomenon was found in *Staphylococcus aureus* by means of which it was no longer susceptible to penicillin. It started producing an enzyme named as penicillinase, which can easily break down the beta lactam ring of penicillin. This ring is necessary to bind bacteria (penicillin binding proteins; PBPs) and therefore its bacterial killing ability. This effect was named as antimicrobial/antibiotic resistance in bacteria. Since then, many different types of bacteria are becoming increasingly resistant to many new antibiotics. The phenomenon of antibiotic resistance in bacteria is a persistently ongoing process and is on rise with every new day. This process can further be increased by humans, e.g., the inappropriate use of antibiotics, following reduced doses of antibiotics than required/standards, using antibiotics as a precautionary measures in viral infections, using antibiotics as growth promoters, prescribing broad-spectrum antibiotics, using antibiotics without using the antimicrobial sensitivity testing, and finally by noncompliance of the animal owner. There has been a surge in the use of antibiotics for treatment of a variety of infections. In fact, nowadays, the use of a variety of anti-infection therapy has become an invaluable tool for the treatment of a variety of bovine infections. Using anti-infective agents has greatly reduced the mortality as well as the morbidity against a variety of microbial infections in animals and humans. However, their frequent use has also led to a major problem in human and animal health, the development of antimicrobial resistance in microbes (ability of a microorganism to tolerate and even grow in the presence of the normal inhibitory concentration), and its transmission to a variety of other microbes (within same or different genera) against these anti-infective agents. The development of the resistance in microbes against anti-infective agents was predictable as the discoverer of the first antibiotic, Dr. Alexander Fleming, discussed this issue in his Nobel prize winning lecture (1945) [2, 3].

The emergence of the antibiotic-resistant strains has been associated with an increased occurrence of the morbidity and mortality by the antibiotic-resistant isolates than caused by the nonresistant isolates in both humans and animals. In the last 6 decades, there has been a tremendous increase in the number of the multidrug-resistant (MDR) isolates in bacterial community, which have been associated with an increase in hospital stay in humans. Nowadays, with an advent of a variety of molecular biology techniques, there have been several mechanisms reported for the development of the resistance in the bacterial populations infecting humans and animals, and this process is ever increasing. Therefore, it is extremely important to know the factors that cause antibiotic resistance in humans and animals, molecular mechanisms of the antimicrobial resistance in different microbes, different methods of the genetic transfer of the resistance among different microbes, and the development of a variety of strategies for the control of bacterial resistance against antimicrobials, so that a better control of the infections in humans as well as in animals can be made.

2. Common bovine infections and their treatment

Currently, in Indo-Pak numerous infectious diseases are prevalent in bovines. Because these are the major source of income for the poor farmers (who merely raise about 4–5 animals), there is massive irregular use of a variety of anti-infectious agents to save their life and thus family earnings. Whereas, in **Table 1**, a list of diseases and their possible treatments in bovines is given.

Infection/disease	Etiology	Treatment options
Hemorrhagic septicemia	*Pasteurella multocida*	Oxytetracycline
Anthrax	*Bacillus anthracis*	Penicillin
Black leg/quarter	*Clostridium chauvoei*	Penicillin
Contagious bovine Pleuropneumonia	*Mycoplasma mycoides*	Tylosin

Table 1. Common bovine infections and their treatment.

3. Factors associated with antimicrobial resistance in animals

Since the discovery of the first antibiotic, penicillin, by Alexander Fleming, there has been a tremendous use of antibiotics in farm animals. In animals, antibiotics have been used as growth promoters as prophylaxis as well as metaphylaxis. Both approaches involve the administration of antibiotics in animals either by injection or through feed/water.

The primary goal of antibiotics was to treat the infectious diseases in animals and, thereby, improve the overall health of animals and humans. However, an unexpected thing observed in chickens during the 1940s was that antibiotic use may also cause an increase in the growth rate in animals. This finding has led to their use as growth promoters. Antibiotics have been used as growth promoters for decades. This aspect is of tremendous controversy since the beginning. The practice employs the use of antibiotics at subtherapeutic levels, with the main purpose to control the enteric and respiratory diseases in farm animals associated with poor management. The exact mechanism by which antibiotic may enhance the growth rate in animals is yet unknown precisely; however, it is postulated that antibiotics may increase the animal growth rate by either one of the following mechanisms:

a. Killing the pathogenic bacterial species in the intestine and thereby reducing the inflammatory conditions

b. Reduced inflammation in the intestinal mucosa leading to the increased absorption of the variety of nutrients from the intestinal tract

c. Increasing the amount of beneficial microbes in the intestinal tract leading to an optimal intestinal environment

d. Synthesis of a variety of bacteriocins (bacterial products made by beneficial bacteria or probiotics which are used to inhibit other pathogenic microbes) and vitamins by the probiotics further increasing animal health

Currently, China, the USA, and Brazil are the leading countries of antibiotic utilization in animals. Approximately, 40 antibiotics have been approved for animals in the USA, out of which more than 30 are currently being used in humans. Majority of antibiotic use in animals falls in either one of the three uses:

3.1. For the treatment of infectious diseases in animals (therapeutic use)

Therapeutic treatment usually involves the treatment of either single or whole herd/flock with specific doses of specific antimicrobial drugs. One typical care should be kept in mind in this aspect is that each animal should receive the complete dose of antibiotics and the antibiotic treatment should be continued for at least 72–120 h. But there may be problems in this aspect of antibiotic use as the diseased animal has greatly reduced appetite, and this thing may lead to the reduced intake of the specific antibacterial drug. This may lead to the potential problem of developing the resistance in microbial communities against these antibiotics [4].

3.2. For the prevention of a variety of infections in animals (prophylactic use)

Traditionally many antibiotics were being used in the feed lot and dairy cattle to prevent against a variety of diseases. However, this practice is discouraged.

3.3. The use of antibiotics as growth promoters

Although the use of antibiotics in animals has greatly contributed in increasing the production in farm animals, however, their use as growth promoter was an issue of great controversy as this practice has greatly enhanced the development of resistance in a variety of microbial species not only in animals but also in humans. Therefore, nowadays, several countries have banned the use of the latest antibiotics as growth promoters in animals (to be intended for human use only in order to minimize the chances for development of antimicrobial resistance) [5, 6].

There are some exceptions in this aspect of development of the resistance in microbial communities against antimicrobial use as AGPs. The typical example is the use of ionophores which are mainly used to reduce the incidence of coccidiosis as well as improve the microbial communities in rumen (favor the microbial communities toward Gram-positive bacteria). Furthermore, latest studies have also shown that the use of the AGPs may contribute toward the disturbance of normal microflora in animals, thereby greatly affecting the immune system of the animals [7–10].

4. Molecular mechanisms of the resistance against major antimicrobial drugs

Although, till now, different types of the resistance mechanisms have been reported in bacteria against different antibiotics, they can be broadly classified as follows.

4.1. Degradation of the antibacterial drug by the bacterial enzymes

Several bacterial beta lactamases can degrade the beta lactam antibiotics. Beta lactamases do it so by degrading the beta lactam ring of the antibiotics. Also, some antibiotics can be degraded by the addition of the specific group, e.g., chloramphenicol molecule possesses hydroxyl group that can be easily acetylated by the incorporation of acetyl-CoA, a reaction that is catalyzed by acetyl transferases. Moreover, aminoglycosides can also be easily degraded by the addition of phosphate, acetyl-CoA, and adenylyl group, and these additions are carried out by the phosphotransferases, acetyl transferases and the adenyl transferases [11, 12].

4.2. Reduced permeability to a drug by bacteria

For example, most of the Gram negatives contain extremely small-sized porin in their outer membrane, and this imparts a major permeability barrier to a large number of antibiotics to cross that barrier. In similar manner, *Mycobacterium* also offers a major permeability barrier to most of the antibiotics as they contain a thick layer of the mycolic acid, and this waxy material hinders the entry of the majority of drugs [13].

4.3. Increased efflux of the drug

Several bacterial species possess the efflux pumps that actively pump out the drug by bacterial cells. Such pumps effectively reduce the bactericidal concentration of a particular antibiotic drug, and they have been actively implicated in the emergence of resistance against a myriad of the antibiotics particularly against tetracyclines, aminoglycosides, and sulfonamides. The examples of bacteria containing these types of pumps include *Pseudomonas, Staphylococcus aureus,* and *E. coli* [14].

4.4. Modification of the drug target

Several drugs act by their initial binding to a particular site within bacterial cells in order to initiate their bactericidal/bacteriostatic activity. So when a drug binding target is changed, it may lead to the development of the resistance in bacteria against that drug. This phenomenon has been incriminated in the emergence of the resistance against antibiotics such as macrolides and phenolics (Chloramphenicol) in which alternations in the binding sites at ribosome drastically reduce the antibacterial activity of these drugs [15].

4.5. Use of an alternative pathway by bacterial cells

Some of the microbes use alternate pathways, and they change the previous pathway which is inhibited by a particular antibiotic. Typical example is that some of the bacteria use the preformed folic acid rather than synthesizing it, which is inhibited by sulfonamides by a phenomenon known as competitive antagonism.

4.6. Specific analysis of antibiotic resistance at molecular level

With an advent of the molecular biology techniques, many mechanisms for the development of antibiotic resistance have been observed in the last half century [2]. One of the major threats nowadays is by the extended spectrum beta lactamases (ESBLs) producing Gram-negative bacteria [11]. Till now, approximately 13,000 different types of the ESBLs have been reported, and they are mainly classified into three different functional groups. Most of the ESBLs are encoded by a gene known as bla, and the most important ones are bla CTX, bla TEM, bla SHV, bla KPC, and bla OXA. One of the major issues is the origin of the carbapenemase enzymes which are mainly associated with the development of the resistance in the carbapenems (e.g., IMP, KPC, VIM beta lactamases, and OXA), major drugs which are used for the treatment of multidrug-resistant (MDR) Gram-negative infections. These enzymes also act on the third- and fourth-generation cephalosporins, e.g., cefquinome and ceftiofur, thus referred as the extended spectrum cephalosporinases (ESCs). One of the major features associated with many ESBLs/ESCs is that they are located in the moveable genetic elements, e.g., plasmids [12]. In similar way, resistance to macrolides is also associated with the development of the resistance in a variety of closely related drugs, i.e., lincosamides, pleuromutilins, and streptogramins, and thus they are referred as PLSA phenotype [16, 17] and MLSB phenotype [18].

Another main point associated with the aminoglycoside resistance is that the same gene in bacteria is responsible for resistance against the gentamicin and apramycin. Moreover it has also been observed that the gene causing the resistance against the aminoglycoside is also responsible for the resistance against the fluoroquinolones [19].

The table below illustrates the different mechanisms of the development of the resistance against a variety of anti-infection drugs used in veterinary medicine. This table clearly depicts that each bacterium possesses a unique set of the resistance mechanisms, and virtually resistance against antibiotics is present in nearly all species. One such example is that the resistance against the macrolide is different in *Staphylococcus* than observed in the *Campylobacter*.

One of the major emerging issues nowadays is the resistance against multiple drugs, i.e., fluoroquinolones and cephalosporins; another such issue is the emerging MDR *E.coli* ST 131 [20, 21]. Some of the old antibiotics, e.g., colistin, which was previously widely used for the control of *E. coli* [21], have been withdrawn so that it may be used to treat a variety of infections caused by the MDR Gram-negative bacterial spp. [22]. However, recently it has been observed in China that bacteria possess the mcr-1 gene which plays an important role in conferring resistance against colistin, and this observation has severely raised questions on the use of colistin for the treatment of a variety of bacterial infections [23–25]. Just immediately afterward, in Belgium, mcr-2 gene was also observed in a bacterium that did not contain the mcr-1 gene and that gene was also responsible for conferring the resistance against colistin in those bacteria [26, 27].

Another important fact is that the emergence of the resistance against one member of a class of antibiotic may result in the development of the resistance against other members of that class. The other mechanism is known as co-selection. This is a phenomenon in which the genes for resistance against a myriad of antibiotics are located in the single plasmid or the mobile genetic element. In this case this mobile genomic element or the plasmid confers the resistance against all the antibiotics. In contrary to this, the other mechanism is that when one bacterium becomes resistant against one microbe, then it exhibits an increased susceptibility against the other antibiotic [28].

4.6.1. Mechanisms of the antibacterial drug resistance

Table 2 illustrates the mechanisms of the bacterial resistance against different drugs. It also depicts various genes involved in the emergence of resistance against that drug.

4.7. Mechanisms of antibacterial resistance transfer in bacteria

One of the major problems is that bacteria not only become resistant to many antibacterial drugs by a variety of phenomena, but they are also capable of transferring this resistance to other bacteria of same as well as with other genera. The main reason for transfer of genetic resistance is because the genes for antibacterial resistance are mainly present on the moveable genomic elements (MGE), e.g., integrons, plasmids, and transposons. But the changes at gene level may also occur in chromosomes although they are extremely rare (except in *Mycobacterium*). This often occurs because there is a change in the drug target and, thus, the antibacterial drug cannot bind to the appropriate binding site, leading to the loss of efficacy of that particular antibiotic. If the use of antibiotics is inappropriate, e.g., not following the well-established dosage regimen for a particular drug against a particular disease, it can dramatically increase the chances of the development of the resistance against that drug because of the selective advantage of changing their genomic elements.

One of the main important locations of antibacterial resistance is the bacterial plasmids. Plasmids are single covalently closed circular pieces of the DNA which are not important in the survival of the bacteria, but they are extremely important in offering an added advantage

Antibiotic class	Members	Target	Resistance mechanism	Genes involved (examples)
Polypeptide	Bacitracin	Cell wall (inhibits peptidoglycan synthesis)	Efflux	Bcr
Tetracycline	Tetracycline Oxytetracycline Chlortetracycline Doxycycline Minocycline	Ribosome (30 S)	Drug efflux Change in binding site Drug modification by bacterial enzymes	Otr, tet
Streptogramins	Virginiamycin	Ribosome	Efflux Change in drug target Drug inactivation by bacterial enzymes	Erm, Isa, Vgb, Vga, cfr, vat
Macrolides	Tylosin Tilmicosin Tiamulin Erythromycin Azithromycin Clarithromycin Spiramycin Tulathromycin	Ribosome (50 S; inhibit the translocation of the aminoacyl tRNA from P site to A site)	Glycosylation Hydrolysis Phosphorylation Efflux Altered drug target	Ere, erm, msr, mef, mph, cfr
Pleuromutilins	Valnemulin	Ribosomes	Altered drug target Efflux of the drug	Sal, cfr, vga, isa
Lincosamides	Lincomycin Clindamycin	Ribosome (50 S; Inhibit the translocation of the aminoacyl tRNA from P site to A site)	Drug efflux Inactivation of the drug Altered drug target	Erm, inu, vga, inu, cfr, msr,
Beta lactams	Penicillin Amoxicillin Ampicillin Cloxacillin Cefuroxime Cefalexin Ceftiofur Cefquinome	Cell wall (inhibit the synthesis of peptidoglycan)	Efflux, Hydrolysis Altered drug target	Ade, mec, bla, mex, cme
Aminoglycosides	Gentamicin Kanamycin Neomycin Apramycin Spiramycin Framycetin	Ribosomes	Inactivation by bacterial enzymes Efflux Altered drug target	Aph, ant, acc, rmt, ade, arm, spd, apw
Fluoroquinolones	Enrofloxacin Marbofloxacin Orbifloxacin Ibafloxacin Pradofloxacin	DNA replication (inhibit the DNA gyrase)	Altered drug target Drug efflux Inactivation of the drug by the bacterial enzymes	Aac (6′), oqx, qnr, gyr A, parC
Phenicols	Florfenicol Chloramphenicol	Ribosomes (50 S; inhibit the peptidyltransferase)	Drug efflux Inactivation of the drug by enzymes Altered drug target	Cat, cfr, cml, flo, optr

Antibiotic class	Members	Target	Resistance mechanism	Genes involved (examples)
Sulfonamides	Sulfamethoxazole	Folic acid synthesis	Altered drug target Increase efflux of the drug	acr, sul
Nitrofurans	Nitrofurazone Nitrofurantoin	DNA	Modification of the target in bacteria Changes in porins	Omp, nfs
Pyrimidines	Trimethoprim	Folic acid synthesis	Modification of the target in bacteria Enhance drug efflux	Dhfr, bpr-opc
Cationic polypeptides	Colistin Polymyxin B	Cell membrane	Modification of the drug target Increased efflux of the drug	pmr AB, mgr

Table 2. Mechanisms of the antibacterial drug resistance.

to the microbes when present. They do it by providing the genes for resistance against many antibacterial drugs. Moreover, they can also make the bacteria resist the toxins and heavy metals. Because of the fact that they are important in providing the bacteria resistance against many factors, that is why they are also called as R factor. Plasmids are extremely important in the development of the resistance against the drugs as they can easily be transferred from one to the other bacteria by means of the pilus. This process is known as conjugation. This process can occur in many species including *Clostridium, E. coli, Bordetella, Salmonella, Proteus, Streptococcus*, and *Shigella*. One important factor should be kept in mind that plasmids may not only be transmitted within a genus but also between genera. This fact is of extreme danger to the bovine as well as public health as resistance in bovine microbial spp. can transfer the resistance in many microbes of public health importance, sometimes even leading to the pandemic spread of the zoonotic and public health pathogens.

However, it should be kept in mind that although the plasmids are often exchanged between bacteria by the process of conjugation, however, they may also be transmitted from one to the other bacteria by means of other methods of genetic transfer, and they may include the transduction and transformation. In transformation, the genetic components of one bacterium are transmitted to the other bacterium when placed in a medium. However, it should be kept in mind that this process is poorly understood, yet at molecular level and moreover, it occurs in limited microbes under specific conditions (the presence of divalent ions or electrical pulses).

Transduction is defined as the transfer of genetic components from one to another bacterium through a bacteriophage (viruses infecting bacteria). When a virus infects the bacterial cells, there is possibility that during integration with the host cell genome, it may take away some components of those bacterial cells in the process when it leaves the cells. Two types of transduction are possible. One is generalized transduction in which any component of the bacterial cell may be transmitted. On the other hand, the specialized transduction is one in which the virus carries only the specific component of the bacterial cells (mostly surrounding portion of the integration site). When the same bacteriophage may infect the other cell, it can transfer the genes of previous bacteria into the new bacteria. The process of transduction occurs with the greatest frequency in gram-positive bacteria.

A single plasmid may carry the genes for antibacterial resistance against many drugs (3–9); thus, the whole population of the bacteria may become multidrug resistant by the process of plasmid transfer although the animals may be treated with only one drug. A single plasmid has been found to carry the genes of antibacterial drug resistance at against least nine different drugs.

Other MGEs may also play an important role in the emergence of antibacterial resistance in microbial populations. Many transposons may also carry the genes for antibacterial drug resistance, and they are rapidly moving within the bacteria leading to the emergence of antibacterial drugs resistance in microbes. Some examples of the transposons include the Tn05 (bleomycin, kanamycin, and streptomycin), Tn21 (spectinomycin, streptomycin, and sulfonamides), and Tn4001 (tobramycin, gentamicin, and kanamycin).

A genetic component that carries many genes against many antibiotics together in the form of gene cassettes is also known as integrons. An integrin is normally a nonreplicating piece of the DNA that is often associated with a plasmid, chromosomes, or integrons. The integrons also play an important role in the spread of antibiotic resistance against many microbes as they are also easily transmitted from one to the other bacterial spp.

4.8. Determination of antibiotic susceptibility

Although antibiotics have been made many years ago, however, still little information is available on how to use antibiotics in which way. Although there are many guidelines about the treatment of specific infections with specific antimicrobial agents, however, still it is often extremely difficult to select an appropriate antibiotic to treat a particular disease. This happens primarily as many factors contribute to the selection of an appropriate antibiotic, and they include animal species affected (some antibiotics are contraindicated in bovine because of public health issues, or they are too much toxic for animals),the infection (aerobic or anaerobic, soft tissue or hard tissue infection), microorganism susceptibility to a particular agent, drug behavior within the body (pharmacodynamics, e.g., where the drug distributes more effec- tively and toxicity profile of the drug within the body), dosage regimen of particular antibiotic, route of administration, and various drug residues. Majority of the mentioned parameters are studied in depth while designing and final approval of the drug, but still pharmacodynamics of a particular drug are often unpredictable in some animals and the site of infection also matters in the selection of antibiotics.

So, testing antimicrobial compounds to determine the antimicrobial susceptibility in various bacteria becomes an extremely important parameter to be determined, before making a final decision about the antibiotic use in animals. On the basis of the results of the antibiotic sensitivity testing, the organisms may be classified as the susceptible, intermediate, or resistant microorganisms. However, an important aspect should be kept in mind that antibiotic is not equally effective against all bacteria even if they belong to the same spp. A typical example is *Pasteurella multocida*, which causes the respiratory infection in bovines. When its (isolated from many animals from different countries) antibiotic susceptibility was done against ampicillin, then different isolates demonstrated different levels of the susceptibility and resistance against the same drug (Penicillins). In addition, it is possible that an antibiotic is initially highly effective in the treatment of a particular infection; however, with the passage of time, its effectiveness may become lower. This problem may arise if the animal is treated many times with the same antibiotic or is exposed to the suboptimal concentration of a particular antibiotic.

So because of this intense variation in antibiotic response against different infections, it becomes imperative to accurately test the antibiotic susceptibility routinely prior to make any decision. The results provided by some of the routinely used antibiotic susceptibility tests can provide some guidance about the susceptibility profile of bacteria against different antibiotics. However, it should also be kept in mind that although these in vitro antibiotic profile may provide us with an idea of bacterial antibiotic susceptibility testing, however, still they do not provide any guarantee to be effective in vivo. A simpler scenario may be that when animals is suffering from an anaerobic infection in which *E. coli* is primarily the causative organisms, in vitro test may show that aminoglycosides possess good antibacterial activity against the *E. coli*; however, if only the interpretation of that result is kept in mind and aminoglycosides are used to threat that infection, there will be treatment failure. This is because of the fact that aminoglycosides need oxygen-based uptake within the bacteria, and in anaerobic environment, there is no uptake of the aminoglycosides leading to the failure of treatment. Similarly, different drugs have different affinities for different tissues, and thus if some drug is unable to reach to a particular tissue, it is unable to demonstrate its microbial killing or inhibition activity. Moreover, nowadays a very hot research issue is how to control bacterial population in biofilms. Different bacteria make biofilms which are collections of millions of the microbes. In biofilms, microbial population becomes extremely resistant to a particular drug, as it does not allow the drug to penetrate the microbial populations. In short various factors are responsible for an antimicrobial drug to demonstrate different antibacterial effects in vitro and in vivo.

Although the assays for the determination of the antimicrobial sensitivity were developed just after the discovery of the first antibiotic, penicillin, however, they were poorly designed assays, and they exhibited a greater variability not only among different communities but within the same hospital. So there was a pressing issue for the development of the test which exhibits greater reproducibility and may be applied universally across the globe. So after a lot of hit and trial method, researcher became successful in devising an assay which is used till now as one of the most preferred methods for the determination of the antibiotic susceptibility testing in microbes. This test was developed by Bauer in 1966 and is known as disk diffusion assay of antimicrobial sensitivity in microbes.

4.8.1. Disk diffusion test for antimicrobial sensitivity

This is one of the most widely assays currently being used in veterinary medicine because this assay can be used to test the antimicrobial activity of many drugs against any bacterial spp., and it is also economical.

The test is based on the use of disk impregnated with antibacterial compound and placing it on the agar plate (Muller Hinton agar) which is cultured with 1×10^8 microorganisms/ml of the suspension. When the antibiotic disk is placed on the agar surface, it allows the antibiotic to move in a lateral position due to diffusion. This results in the generation of the antibiotic gradient along the agar surface. Near the antibiotic disk, the concentration of the antibiotic is higher, but as the distance increases from the disk, it causes a reduced concentration of the antibiotic. This results in the production of the zone of inhibition of the bacterial growth. This zone gives an indirect idea for the estimation of the minimum inhibitory concentration of the drug that is required against particular bacterium.

The disk diffusion method can also be affected by many different types of factors. The first one is the thickness of the agar in the petri plate. The recommended thickness of agar medium is 4 mm. If the thickness of the agar medium is more than the recommended thickness, it will result in the reduced diffusion of the drug in lateral direction, resulting in false interpretation of the antimicrobial sensitivity test. If the thickness of the plate is less than the recommended thickness, it will result in increased drug diffusion in the lateral direction. The second factor is the bacterial concentration. If the bacterial concentration in the media is less than the recommended, it will result in an increased zone of inhibition, which leads to the false interpretation of the test. Similarly, if the concentration of the bacterial suspension is more than the standard one, it will also mislead the final interpretation. If the generation time of the microorganism is too long, e.g., *Arcanobacterium*, it will result in an increased zone of inhibition leading to a false interpretation. Another factor to be kept in mind while conducting antibiotic sensitivity testing is the placement of the disks on agar. The standard distance is 24 mm. If the distance is too small between two antibiotic disks, it may lead to overlap among various zones of inhibition making the interpretation of the assay difficult.

One major disadvantage of this test is that this assay is mainly qualitative. Although it gives us an idea about the minimum inhibitory concentration of a particular drug against a particular microbe, however, still it is one of the most commonly used particularly in developing countries, where infrastructure is poor at local veterinary hospitals. The other advantage of this test is that it is an extremely simpler test to carry out with a minimum cost. The results of this assay are available within 24–48 h for most of the bacterial pathogens of bovine importance [29].

4.8.2. E-test

The other method of determination of antibiotic sensitivity is the E-test. The disadvantage of the disk diffusion assay can be mitigated by using another similar test which almost involves the same technique; however, it gives a nearly realistic value of the MIC of particular antibiotics against a particular bacterium. The test is named as E-test.

The principle of the E-test is based on the lateral diffusion of the drug from a plastic strip which is impregnated with the different conc. of the antibiotics usually starting from 0. Along the length of the plastic strip, the concentration of the antibiotic increases gradually, thus creating a continuous gradient of antibiotic concentration along the plastic strip.

So at the beginning where the concentration of antibiotic is zero, there is usually no zone of the inhibition. As the concentration of the antibiotic increases, there is a proportional increase in the zone of inhibition around the plastic strip.

Although E-test gives us quantity data regarding the MIC against a particular bacterium, however, it is expensive to carry out, which makes it difficult to be carried out under field conditions; however, it may be used for research purpose against a particular bacterium [30].

4.9. Strategies to reduce the antimicrobial resistance

As development of antibiotic resistance in major microbes is posing a major threat to animal and human populations, it requires efforts at gross root level to reduce this problem. Several different strategies may be adopted which are extremely important for the reduction in the emergence of antibacterial resistance. This may involve the early detection and diagnosis of the infectious diseases, the use of alternatives to antibiotics, estimation of the cost and relative benefit analysis, and using immunomodulation.

4.9.1. Early detection and diagnosis of diseases

This strategy may also aid a lot in the reduction of antimicrobial use and thus develop resistance as discussed; see [29]. Several diseases have different parameters, which may give an important indicator about the disease occurrence at an earlier stage. For example, several liver enzymes and kidney enzymes start to alter their serum conc. And this may provide an initial indicator for a variety of infectious diseases at earlier stages. Several infectious diseases produce systemic indicators, such as increase in the serum proteins, and this effect is collectively known as acute phase response to an infection. In acute phase response, several acute phase proteins are greatly increased in their serum concentration. Similarly at initial stages of viral and bacterial infection, there are changes in the conc. of the specific cytokines in the serum of an animal. All of these acute phase proteins and changes in the levels of the different cytokines can easily be detected by a variety of laboratory tests (e.g., ELISA). Although this approach requires a state-of-the-art diagnostic laboratory facility, using this approach can help in the reduction of the emergence of the antibiotic residues in bovines. All of these changes in earlier stages of infection are the consequences of systemic inflammatory response which can easily be controlled by the use of a variety of anti-inflammatory drugs, i.e., nonsteroidal anti-inflammatory drugs. This treatment can be augmented by using the strategy of nutritional modulation in dairy animals by supplementing feed with omega-3 fatty acid, phytochemicals (e.g., *Aloe arborescence*, *Echinacea purpurea*), and antioxidants. It has been observed that using this strategy can lead to the reduction in the incidence of many reproductive diseases, ketosis, and somatic cell count in milk.

The above strategy may be adopted with a greatest success in terms of the reduction of the antibiotics use in animals, but this strategy also necessitates the routinely strict monitoring and inspection of the dairy herd. A variety of animal welfare and health parameters should be regularly monitored, and they include recording the dry matter intake of animals, milk somatic cell count, rectal temperature, the presence of blood or fibrin clots in milk, and noting any teat lesions. It has been observed that routine monitoring of these parameters can result in earlier detection of the disease and therefore earlier and simpler treatments, often not requiring antibiotics (e.g., by improving the ruminal activity with the use of yeast or glucogenic supplementation).

4.9.2. Using antibiotic alternatives

Recently, it has been proposed in the international OIE conference that an emphasis should be placed on the use of antibacterial drug alternatives such as bacteriophages, biological response modifiers (BMRs), antibacterial peptides of natural origin, prebiotics, probiotics, and the use of proper vaccination schedule in animals (given in the table below); probiotics, prebiotics, and BRMs are responsible for the development of the optimal intestinal microbial flora which can overall improve the animal health along with reducing the incidence of the several infectious diseases in dairy animals; see [31–33]. Bacteriophages are extremely specific in infecting particular bacteria, and that is why they pose a minimum toxicity danger in humans and animals, yet this approach is mainly on theoretical grounds and needs many successful clinical trials and intensive knowledge before they may be adapted in animals for treating infectious diseases. Similarly following an appropriate vaccination program in animals (keeping in view of the serotype/strain of the agent to be used in a particular area) can dramatically reduce the occurrence of many primary as well as secondary infections in bovines.

Table 3 illustrates a variety of diseases and their treatment.

Vaccinating the bovine against many infectious diseases can definitely reduce the incidence of majority of bacterial and viral infections, thereby further reducing the usage of the antimicrobials in bovine.

Similarly, using a variety of phytochemicals may also be useful in the treatment of variety of infections. These chemicals derived from different plants act systemically for the treatment of diseases.

For treating the infections of gastrointestinal tract, *Allium sativum* stem is crushed, is boiled in the water, and then is provided to the animals. Its effect is mainly due to the compound present in it also known as allicin which is well known for its antibacterial activity [34, 35]. Also *Cassia fistula* is also being used in treating a variety of GIT maladies of bovines; particularly, it is effective in treating *E. coli* infections effectively. This activity may be due to the presence of several compounds of pharmacological importance including terpenoids, saponins, steroids, anthraquinone, phenolic compounds, and steroids present in them [36]. Similarly seeds of the *Foeniculum vulgare* are mixed with the root of *Glycyrrhiza glabra*, and they are also used to treat the GIT infections [37, 38]. *Morus alba* leaves are given to the animals for

Brucellosis (breeding animals)	4–12 months of age
Vibriosis (breeding animals)	Before breeding
Leptospirosis (breeding animals)	Before breeding
Black leg	March
Anthrax	February–August
Hemorrhagic septicemia	June–December
Foot-and-mouth disease	March–September

Table 3. Vaccination schedule of bovine.

5 days in order to treat constipation. This anticonstipation activity is mainly reported because of the presence of the quercetin, rutin, and apigenin [39, 40]. *Punica granatum* peel has also demonstrated its activity against majority of the GIT pathogens which may be because of the presence of the flavonoids and phenolic compounds in it [41].

One of the most economically devastating diseases of bovine, mastitis, can also be treated by using a variety of phytochemicals. Here again, *Allium sativum* is also routinely being used in the treatment of mastitis. It has shown promising results even against those pathogens which are resistant to many antibiotics [42]. *Zingiber officinale* is also being used to control mastitis in dairy animals [43]. Similarly, *Allium cepa* and *Trachyspermum ammi* mixture was also being routinely used to control mastitis successfully in dairy herds [44].

Bovine often do suffer from a myriad of respiratory infections particularly when kept in a closed humid confinement in winter season and with poor ventilation. Again some compounds are extremely useful in treating respiratory diseases of animals, and they include *Glycyrrhiza glabra* (stem) and *Hordeum vulgare* (seeds). Both of these plants possess a variety of compounds such as saponins, volatile compounds, tannins, and alkaloids which are beneficial in treating a variety of mild to moderate respiratory infections (when treated for 5–7 days) [45, 46].

Similarly for the treatment of a variety of bovine skin infections, many compounds are routinely used, and they include *Aloe barbadensis* leaves (given orally alone or mixing with salts), *Tamarix aphylla* leaves (applied topically), *Citrullus colocynthis* (extracts from fruit and seed), and *Azadirachta indica* (leaves). All of these plants are extremely useful in treating a variety of inflammatory/infectious diseases of bovine skin [47–49].

4.9.3. Estimation of the cost and relative benefit analysis

Although currently there is a great emphasis on the reduction of antibiotic use in animals, however, its use is still needed in some cases of infectious diseases. But in such cases, it is better to prioritize the basis of cost of antibiotics in animals and the benefits achieved. For example, in the case of mastitis, treatment efficacy with the help of gram-negative bacteria depends on several factors including the bacterial spp. involved and the acuteness or chronicity of the disease. Some cases have good outcomes following treatment, while the treatment of the chronically affected animals is often futile. Similarly, some bacterial spp., e.g., *Streptococcus agalactiae* and *Staphylococcus aureus*, along with coagulase-negative *Staphylococcus aureus*, are extremely difficult to treat. This also implies that culturing of the mastitis-infected milk along with antibiotic susceptibility testing should be a routine practice while treating the animals; see [50].

Similarly if the animal is repeatedly suffering from clinical mastitis, particularly after the third lactation, then mostly cost of the treatment becomes extremely higher than the benefits.

4.9.4. Immunomodulator use

Animals often suffer from chronic stress when their welfare is compromised. Stress may be in the form of overcrowding, nutritional deficiency, poor ventilation and temperature control, transportation, and high production. Under stress body physiology is altered, and it results in secretion of cortisol from the adrenal cortex. Under the influence of the adrenal cortisol, the body immune system is greatly compromised. This predisposes the animals to a variety of infectious diseases. So it is better to use immunomodulators in animals under the conditions of stress. This strategy has been discussed in detail; see [51, 52]. These immunomodulators may include the use of vitamins A, C, and E along with minerals such as selenium, copper, and many other minerals. This can dramatically reduce the incidence of many infectious diseases in dairy animals leading toward a reduced use of antibiotics in animals.

5. Conclusion

There are numerous aspects of antibiotic resistance in animals, which are important public health threats for humans, and therefore it is imperative to make as many possible efforts to reduce the emergence of antibiotic resistance in farm animals. It may involve maintaining the animal welfare and good nutritional and immunological status, routine examination of the herd, early detection and appropriate diagnosis of infectious diseases in animals, appropriate therapy at time and the use of antibiotic alternatives such as bacteriophages and vaccination, the use of phenomena of competitive exclusion (by using pre-, pro-, and synbiotics), biological response modifiers, and appropriate immunomodulation in animals. Implementing such programs at national level requires huge financial and political support for ongoing efforts to effectively control the emergence of antibacterial resistance in major bacterial spp. Although using these approaches may not completely assure the avoidance of antibiotics and, therefore, the possibility of emergence of antibiotics, yet, these approaches may aid in slowing down the antibiotic resistance to a greater extent in animals leading toward a great step in improving the public health.

Conflict of interest

Authors have no conflict of interest.

Author details

Muhammad Ashraf[1], Behar-E-Mustafa[2], Shahid-Ur-Rehman[3], Muhammad Khalid Bashir[1]* and Muhammad Adnan Ashraf[4]

*Address all correspondence to: mkhalidbashir@uaf.edu.pk

1 Animal Breeding and Genetics, University of Agriculture, Faisalabad, Pakistan

2 Microbiology, University of Agriculture, Faisalabad, Pakistan

3 Molecular Biology, University of Agriculture, Faisalabad, Pakistan

4 Institute of Microbiology, University of Agriculture, Faisalabad, Pakistan

References

[1] Tampa M, Sarbu I, Matei C, Benea V, Georgescu S. Brief history of syphilis. Journal of Medicine and Life. 2014;**7**:4-10

[2] Davies J, Davies D. Origins and evolution of antibiotic resistance. Microbiology and Molecular Biology Reviews: MMBR. 2010;**74**:417-433. DOI: 10.1128/MMBR.00016-10

[3] Frankel RB, Kalmijn AJ, Amann R, Ludwig W, Petersen N, Arakaki A, Matsunaga T, Bleil U, Kirschvink JL, Siever SM. Sampling the antibiotic resistome. Science. 2006;**311**:374-378

[4] Apley M, Bush E, Morriso R, Singer R, Snelson H. Use estimates of in-feed antimicrobials in swine production in the United States. Foodborne Pathogens and Disease. 2012;**9**:272-279. DOI: 10.1089/fpd.2011.0983

[5] Roy-Chowdhury P, McKinnon J, Wyrsch E, Hammond J, Charles I, Djordjevic S. Genomic interplay in bacterial communities: Implications for growth promoting practices in animal husbandry. Frontiers in Microbiology. 2014;**5**:394. DOI: 10.3389/fmicb.2014.00394

[6] Sandegren L. Selection of antibiotic resistance at very low antibiotic concentrations. Upsala Journal of Medical Sciences. 2014;**119**:103-107

[7] Nobel Y, Cox L, Kirigin F, Bokulich N, Yamanishi S, Teitler I, Chung J, Sohn J, Barber C, Goldfarb D, Raju K, Abubucker S, Zhou Y, Ruiz V, Li H, Mitreva M, Alekseyenko A, Weinstock G, Sodergren E, Blaser M. Metabolic and metagenomic outcomes from early-life pulsed antibiotic treatment. Nature Communications. 2015;**6**:7486. DOI: 10.1038/ncomms8486

[8] Schulfer A, Blaser M. Risks of antibiotic exposures early in life on the developing microbiome. PLoS Pathogens. 2015;**11**:1004903. DOI: 10.1371/journal.ppat.1004903

[9] Holman D, Chénier M. Temporal changes and the effect of subtherapeutic concentrations of antibiotics in the gut microbiota of swine. FEMS Microbiology Ecology. 2014;**90**:599-608

[10] Looft T, Allen H, Cantarel B, Levine U, Bayles D, Alt D, Henrissat B, Stanton T. Bacteria, phages and pigs: The effects of in-feed antibiotics on the microbiome at different gut locations. The ISME Journal. 2014;**8**:1566-1576. DOI: 10.1038/ismej.2014.12

[11] Rubin J, Pitout J. Extended-spectrum β-lactamase, carbapenemase and AmpC producing *Enterobacteriaceae* in companion animals. Veterinary Microbiology. 2014;**170**:10-18. DOI: 10.1016/j.vetmic.2014.01.017

[12] Trott D. β-lactam resistance in Gram-negative pathogens isolated from animals. Current Pharmaceutical Design. 2013;**19**:239-249

[13] Pages JM, James CE, Winterhalter M. The porin and the permeating antibiotic: A selective diffusion barrier in Gram-negative bacteria. Nature Reviews. Microbiology. 2008;**6**:893-903. DOI: 10.1038/nrmicro1994

[14] Brincat JP, Carosati E, Sabatini S, Manfroni G, Fravolini A, Raygada JL. Discovery of novel inhibitors of the NorA multidrug transporter of *Staphylococcus aureus*. Journal of Medicinal Chemistry. 2011;**54**:354-365. DOI: 10.1021/jm1011963

[15] Spratt BG. Resistance to antibiotics mediated by target alterations. Science (New York, N.Y.). 1994;**264**:388-393

[16] Lambert T. Antibiotics that affect the ribosome. Revue Scientifique et Technique. 2012;**31**: 57-64

[17] Zhang A, Xu C, Wang H, Lei C, Liu B, Guan Z, Yang C, Yang Y, Peng L. Presence and new genetic environment of pleuromutilin-lincosamide-streptogramin A resistance gene lsa(E) in *Erysipelothrix rhusiopathiae* of swine origin. Veterinary Microbiology. 2015;**177**:162-167. DOI: 10.1016/j.vetmic.2015.02.014

[18] Hao H, Cheng G, Iqbal Z, Ai X, Hussain H, Huang L, Dai M, Wang Y, Liu Z, Yuan Z. Benefits and risks of antimicrobial use in food-producing animals. Frontiers in Microbiology. 2014;**5**:288. DOI: 10.3389/fmicb.2014.00288

[19] Mathers A, Peirano G, Pitout J. The role of epidemic resistance plasmids and international high-risk clones in the spread of multidrug-resistant *Enterobacteriaceae*. Clinical Microbiology Reviews. 2015;**28**:565-591. DOI: 10.1128/CMR.00116-14

[20] Nicolas-Chanoine M, Bertrand X, Madec J. *Escherichia coli* ST131, an intriguing clonal group. Clinical Microbiology Reviews. 2014;**27**:543-574. DOI: 10.1128/CMR.00125-13

[21] Rhouma M, Beaudry F, Letellier A. Resistance to colistin: What is the fate for this antibiotic in pig production? International Journal of Antimicrobial Agents. 2016;**48**:119-126. DOI: 10.1016/j.ijantimicag.2016.04.008

[22] Theuretzbacher U, Van Bambeke F, Cantón R, Giske C, Mouton J, Nation R, Paul M, Turnidge J, Kahlmeter G. Reviving old antibiotics. The Journal of Antimicrobial Chemotherapy. 2015;**70**:2177-2181. DOI: 10.1093/jac/dkv157

[23] Bialvaei A, Samadi Kafil H. Colistin. Mechanisms and prevalence of resistance. Current Medical Research and Opinion. 2015;**31**:707-721. DOI: 10.1185/03007995.2015.1018989

[24] Catry B, Cavaleri M, Baptiste K, Grave K, Grein K, Holm A, Jukes H, Liebana E, Navas A, Mackay D, Magiorakos A, Romo M, Moulin G, Madero C, Pomba M, Powell M, Pyörälä S, Rantala M, Ružauskas M, Sanders P, Teale C, Threlfall E, Törneke K, van Duijkeren E, Edo J. Use of colistin-containing products within the European Union and European Economic Area (EU/EEA): Development of resistance in animals and possible impact on human and animal health. International Journal of Antimicrobial Agents. 2015;**46**(3):297-306. DOI: 10.1016/j.ijantimicag.2015.06.005

[25] Liu YY, Wang Y, Walsh TR, Yi LX, Zhang R, Spencer J, Doi Y, Tian G, Dong B, Huang X, Yu LF, Gu D, Ren H, Chen X, Lv L, He D, Zhou H, Liang Z, Liu JH, Shen J. Emergence of plasmid-mediated colistin resistance mechanism MCR-1 in animals and human beings in China: A microbiological and molecular biological study. The Lancet Infectious Diseases. 2015;**16**:161-168. DOI: 10.1016/S1473-3099(15)00424-7

[26] Al-Tawfiq JA, Laxminarayan R, Mendelson M. How should we respond to the emergence of plasmid-mediated colistin resistance in humans and animals? International Journal of Infectious Diseases. 2016;**54**:77-84. DOI: 10.1016/j.ijid.2016.11.415

[27] Xavier BB, Lammens C, Butaye P, Goossens H, Malhotra-Kumar S. Complete sequence of an IncFII plasmid harbouring the colistin resistance gene mcr-1 isolated from Belgian pig farms. The Journal of Antimicrobial Chemotherapy. 2016;**71**:2342-2344. DOI: 10.1093/jac/dkw191

[28] Cantón R, Ruiz-Garbajos P. Co-resistance: An opportunity for the bacteria and resistance genes. Current Opinion in Pharmacology. 2011;**11**:477-485. DOI: 10.1016/j.coph.2011.07.007

[29] Trevisi E, Picciolo Cappelli F, Cogrossi S, Grossi P. Administration of an homogenate of *Aloe arborescense* to periparturient dairy cows: Effect on energy metabolism and inflammatory status. Italian Journal of Animal Science. 2013;**82**:1664-1670

[30] Rennie R, Turnbull L, Brosnikoff C. Comparison of Oxoid M.I.C. Evaluator device with broth microdilution and E test device from AB Biodisk for antimicrobial susceptibility testing of *Enterobacteriaceae* [abstract P859]. In: Program and Abstracts of the 18th Annual Meeting of the European Congress on Clinical Microbiology and Infectious Diseases, Barcelona; European Congress on Clinical Microbiology and Infectious Diseases; 2008

[31] Frola I, Pellegrino M, Espeche MC, Larriestra A, Nader-Macias ME, Bogni C. Effect of inflammatory inoculation of *Lactobacillus perolens* CRL1724 in lactating cow udders. Journal of Dairy Research. 2012;**79**:84-92. DOI: 10.1017/S0022029911000835

[32] Loor JJ, Bertoni G, Hosseini A, Roche JR, Trevisi E. Functional welfare using biochemical and molecular technologies to understand better the welfare state of peripartal dairy cattle. Animal Production Science. 2013;**53**:931-953

[33] Trevisi E, Amadori M, Cogrossi S, Razzuoli E, Bertoni G. Metabolic stress and inflammatory response in high yielding periparturient dairy cows. Research in Veterinary Science. 2012;**93**:695-704. DOI: 10.1016/j.rvsc.2011.11.008

[34] Cavallito CJ, Bailey JH. Allicin, the antibacterial principle of *Allium sativum*. I. Isolation, physical properties and antibacterial action. Journal of the American Chemical Society. 1944;**66**:1950-1951

[35] Saravanan P, Ramya V, Sridhar H, Balamurugan V, Umamaheshwari S. Antibacterial activity of *Allium sativum L.* on pathogenic bacterial strains. Global Veterinaria. 2010;**4**:519-522

[36] Bhalodia NR, Nariya PB, Acharya RN, Shukla VJ. In vitro antibacterial and antifungal activities of *Cassia fistula Linn.* fruit pulp extracts. AYU. 2012;**33**:123-129

[37] Manonmani R, Mohideen V, Khadir A. Antibacterial screening of *Foeniculum vulgare Mill.* International Journal of Pharma and Bio Sciences. 2011;**2**:390-394

[38] Nitalikar MM, Munde KC, Dhore BV, Shikalgar SN. Studies of antibacterial activities of *Glycyrrhiza glabra* root extract. International Journal of PharmTech Research. 2010;**2**:899-901

[39] Devi B, Sharma N, Kumar D, Jeet K. *Morus alba* Linn: A phytopharmacological review. International Journal of Pharmacy and Pharmaceutical Sciences. 2013;**5**:14-18

[40] Doi K, Kojima T, Makino M, Kimura Y, Fujimoto Y. Studies on the constituents of the leaves of *Morus alba* L. Chemical and Pharmaceutical Bulletin. 2001;**49**:151-153

[41] Al-Zoreky NS. Antimicrobial activity of pomegranate (*Punica granatum* L.) fruit peels. International Journal of Food Microbiology. 2009;**134**:244-248. DOI: 10.1016/j.ijfoodmicro.2009.07.002

[42] Dilshad SMR, Rehman NU, Ahmad N, Iqbal A. Documentation of ethnoveterinary practices for mastitis in dairy animals in Pakistan. Pakistan Veterinary Journal. 2010;**30**:167-171

[43] Poeloengan M. The effect of red ginger (*Zingiber officinale Roscoe*) extract on the growth of mastitis causing bacterial isolates. African Journal of Microbiology Research. 2011;**5**:382-389

[44] Fujisawa H, Watanabe K, Suma K. Antibacterial potential of garlic-derived allicin and its cancellation by sulfhydryl compounds. Bioscience, Biotechnology, and Biochemistry. 2009;**73**:1948-1955

[45] Kushwah P, Vir DK, Kayande N, Patidar R. Phytochemical screening and Evaluation of antimicrobial activity of *Glycyrrhiza glabra* Linn. PharmaTutor. 2014;**2**:144-147

[46] Jebor AM, Al-Saadi A, Behjet RH, Al-Terehi M, Zaidan HK, Mohammed AK. Characterization and antimicrobial activity of barley grain (*Hordeum vulgare*) extract. International Journal of Current Microbiology and Applied Sciences. 2013;**2**:41-48

[47] Devraj A, Karpagam T. Evaluation of anti-inflammatory activity and analgesic effect of *Aloe vera* leaf extract in rats. International Research Journal of Pharmacy. 2011;**2**:103-110

[48] Yadav SS, Bhukal RK, Bhandoria MS, Ganie SA, Gulia SK, Raghav TBS. Ethnoveterinary medicinal plants of Tosham block of district Bhiwani (Haryana) India. Journal of Applied Pharmaceutical Science. 2014;**4**:40-48. DOI: 10.7324/JAPS.2014.40606

[49] Marzouk B, Marzouk Z, Fenina N, Bouraoui A, Aouni M. Anti-inflammatory and analgesic activities of *Tunisian Citrullus colocynthis Schrad.* immature fruit and seed organic extracts. European Review for Medical and Pharmacological Sciences. 2011;**15**:665-672

[50] Zecconi A. La mastitie bovina: Epidemiologia e costi della patologia. La Settimana Veterinaria. 2013;**849**:4-32. (in Italian)

[51] Amadori M, Stefanon B, Sgorion S, Farinacci M. Immune system response to stress factors. Italian Journal of Animal Science. 2009;**8**:287-299. DOI: 10.4081/ijas.2009.s1.287

[52] Zecconi A, Piccinini R, Fiorina S, Cabrini L, Dapra V, Amador M. Evaluation of interleukin-2 treatment for the prevention of inflammatory infections in cows after calving. Comparative Immunology, Microbiology and Infectious Diseases. 2009;**32**:439-451

Chapter 5

Meat Quality of Indonesian Local Cattle and Buffalo

Henny Nuraini, Edit Lesa Aditia and
Bram Brahmantiyo

Additional information is available at the end of the chapter

http://dx.doi.org/10.5772/intechopen.79904

Abstract

Indonesia have alot of indigenous of cattle breed that already adapted with local condition like bali cattle, madura cattle, ongole crossbred cattle, sumba ongole, aceh cattle and other. The purpose of this review was to determine the quality of meat from local cattle and buffalo in Indonesia. Livestock products in Indonesia must follow ASUH rules that are Aman (safe), Sehat (healthy), Utuh (Wholesomeness) and Halal. Halal food is food that is free from any components that Muslims are prohibited to consuming. The critical point of halal to the product of animal origin is the animal species, the slaughtering process, the distribution until the process of preparing the product for the consumer. Local beef cattle and buffalo meats were more red, tough (warner bratzler shear force > 4.6 kgcm^{-2}), low flavor (marbling, texture and juiceness) than imported meat. Some of the circumstances causing the low quality of meat in Indonesia are most of the breeders employing cattle and buffalo, low quality of feeding, older slaughter age and handling before and at the time of slaughtering process that does not pay attention to aspects of animal welfare. Efforts to improve livestock management, selection and crosses with *Bos taurus* breeds.

Keywords: meat quality, local cattle, buffalo, meat tenderness, muscle microstructure

1. Introduction

Local livestock is crossing cattle or introduction from outside that has been bred in Indonesia until the fifth or more generation has adapted to the local environment and/or management (the Law No. 18/2009 on Husbandry and Animal Health). Indonesian local cattle include bali cattle, ongole crossbreed cattle, madura cattle, sumba ongole, aceh cattle and others, as well as buffalo marshes and river buffalo. The main source of meat in Indonesia comes from local cattle and buffalo, and beef is a livestock commodity that became the main source of animal protein and became one of the main foodstuffs in Indonesia.

The population of cattle in 2017 is 16,599,247 head and buffalo only about 1,395,191 head. Bali cattle is the breed cattle with the highest population when compared with other cattle such as ongole cattle, ongole crossbreed (PO) cattle, aceh cattle, pasundan and madura cattle. Farmer's demand on bali cattle are great because they have many benefits, such as having high reproduction efficiency, fast breeding, potential in producing meat with high carcass percentage and also have a good adaptability to the environment.

Ref. [1] reported that Kebumen district is feasible to be a source of PO cattle breeding because the reproduction of PO cattle in this area is good enough and its population dynamics are expected to increase from 2015 to 2019. Local ciamis cattle have carcass percentage which is not different from Bali cattle, PO and crosses cattle. Local ciamis cattle have a closer genetic distance to PO cattle [2]. Each area has a specific cattle breed, such as Aceh, West Sumatra (pesisir cattle), West Java (pasundan cattle), and the breed's wider spread is a bali cattle and ongole cross breed cattle. In addition, the potential of buffalo in several regions of Indonesia, such as Banten, West Sumatra, Demak, West Nusa Tenggara also make this livestock as a source of meat in Indonesia [3].

The diversity of local feeds in Indonesia also creates different feed quality between regions. Agricultural areas produce agricultural waste that can be used as a source of feed [4]. The use of sorghum silage in cattle fattening could increase meat production by 12.7% with the best growth response achieved by ongole crossbreed cattle. Several other studies also suggest that local cattle provide a rapid growth response through the fattening process [5–7]. The research results showed that local cattle (sumba ongole) with high energy rations have a weight of life and value higher marbling, and more efficient use of ration compared to low energy and medium energy ration. Production performance and quality of local beef can be improved through fattening with rations high energy [6]. To meet the needs of meat and improve the quality of local beef, Indonesia also imports several breeds such as brahman cross, simmental, limousine and angus. The imported cattle have adapted well, even crossed with local cattle in order to improve the quality of meat [8].

Indonesia with a variety of ethnic, cultural and custom has a variety of cuisine based on meat cooked by the method of wet cooking. Wet cooking methods in Indonesia are grouped into several techniques that used the basic ingredients of water to cook it. Wet cooking techniques are boiling, poaching, braising, stewing, simmering, and steaming. This cooking technique actually adjusts to the quality of meat in the market. Beef or buffalo derived from local livestock is generally less tender so it is suitable with wet cooking techniques.

Application of the concept of quality at this time is very important, so that the resulting product can compete in domestic and foreign trade. The term quality means fitness for use [9]. The definition is universal that can be applied to all types of goods and services. The concept is oriented to the assessment or views of consumers as users of goods or services. If the goods produced by the manufacturer match or in accordance with the wishes of consumers, then the goods or services have a good sale value. According to [10] the definition of meat quality is a measure of the characteristics or characteristics of meat assessed by consumers.

The quality of the meat is a special part of the quality of production (production quality) and should clearly be distinguished from the quality of production. The assessment of carcass composition is one part of the quality of production, although it may be a factor influencing the quality of meat. The ecological and animal welfare aspects are part of the quality of production [11]. Furthermore, these factors can be categorized into factors prior to slaughter and factors after slaughter. The assessment of meat quality is an attempt to predict the nature of palatability, processing and cooking of meat. The nature of palatability of meat means acceptable ingredients of meat (fits) with the senses of the eyes, nose and ears [12]. Indonesia's condition with tropical climate, unstable feed quality and traditional rearing management caused the quality of beef and buffalo not to compete in the international market [13]. This situation creates two different meat markets in Indonesia, that is, traditional markets and specific markets (for hotel, restaurant and catering).

The purpose of this review was to determine the quality of local beef and buffalo meat in Indonesia.

2. Meat quality

The quality of meat is a special part of a product quality that is a combination of several important factors when it comes to using the product. When described in an equation, the quality of meat [11] is:

$$Q = \Sigma \, fi \, . \, xi \tag{1}$$

where: Q = quality; f = weighting of the assessed factors from 0 to 1; x = the factor itself.

What matters is the assessment and determining factors are different for each person and also depend on the purpose of performing a quality assessment.

The quality of production will affect the quality of the product such as the occurrence of DFD (dark, firm, dry), hygiene of the slaughter process and aging after the post mortem process. Production quality also affects judgments, for example, from ecological aspects, such as religion, ethnicity and ethics, are currently receiving much attention from consumers. Indonesia has the largest Muslim consumer, so the religious aspect of halal meat is very important.

Assessment of nutritional aspects, as part of hygiene indicators and some technological factors such as pH or myofibril protein content can be measured by chemical analysis. Microbiological aspects as part of hygiene indicators can be evaluated by indicators such as ATP and pyruvate detection or cell differentiation and cell counting. Technological characteristics can be measured physically such as water holding capacity and shear force to measure tenderness. Sensory assessment is a very difficult part to measure in meat quality assessment, this is because it involves the factor of subjectivity in the assessment.

Briefly it can be mentioned that the quality of production and product quality consists of several factors that can be described and measured objectively, where the quality of production affects product quality. While the assessment is a subjective illustration to determine the likes or dislikes by consumers. The description illustrates that the quality of meat is a combination of several assessments and could be divided into:

1. religious aspect

2. sensory quality

3. nutritional quality

4. hygienic and toxicological quality

5. technological quality

Factors affecting of meat quality characteristics can be classified on the physical and chemical properties of meat (called internal factors = internal determinants/IDs) and external factors of meat or livestock. Some internal factors have a direct influence on the characteristics of meat quality (e.g. the concentration of myoglobin affects the color of the meat). However, for some of its indirect effects. For example, two important livestock characteristics, namely genotype and sex are internal factors, but their effect on quality through indirect media.

Internal factors that affect the quality of meat can be divided into primary and secondary internal factors, depend on direct or indirect influence. Primary internal factors such as connective tissue, muscle fiber size, mixed muscle fiber types, concentration and muscle glycogen content, degree of fat and adipose tissue composition. Secondary internal factors include solubility and collagen concentration, metabolic characteristics, muscle ultimate pH, myoglobin form, degree of muscle contraction, fat pigment level, fatty acid proportion. But in reality, the relationship between these factors can occur more than two or three aspects. Changes in meat quality patterns can be estimated due to the growth process. Besides, the influence of other factors such as genotype and nutrition will also affect the pattern of change.

Other factors that affect the quality of meat are external factors. External factors are technical factors as how to handle livestock before, during and after the slaughtering process. Handling or treatment before livestock is slaughter, duration of resting and fasting of livestock. Furthermore, the process of slaughter, electrical stimulation and aging/chilling process will have a lot of effect on the quality of meat.

3. Quality of Indonesian local meat

In this section we will describe the quality of Indonesian local cattle and buffalo, both qualitative and quantitative. Livestock products in Indonesia must follow ASUH rules that are Aman (safe),

Sehat (healthy), Utuh (Wholesomeness) and Halal. To meet the needs of domestic meat, local beef and buffalo showed the same quality as beef crossbreed cattle [14]. The results showed that physical and chemical quality of local beef cattle (ongole grade) was not different from cross-breed cattle. Independent *t* test was no different for the variable: water content, protein content, fat content, pH, WHC and texture. However, other researchers reported that the slaughter weight of the Bali cattle and Madura cattle are generally below average (270.30 ± 63.07 kg) of optimal slaughter weight, so the productivity of cattle with this small frame size is still low, preferably small frame size beef cattle is slaughter if the level of body fatness is fat [15]. Slaughter weight of Madura cattle to meet the traditional market demand is 338.07 kg [13] and Bali cattle which is intensively fattened, able to achieve slaughter weight 343.017 kg [5].

3.1. Religion aspects

Islam as religion has a quality criterion for a very important product that is halal. Halal food is food that is free from any components that Muslims are prohibited to consuming. The growing awareness of Muslim consumers about their religious obligations is halal food, creating greater demand for halal food and other consumer goods. Indonesia is currently a potential market for halal food considering that over 80% of the population is Muslim. Halal meat is one of the products that should receive special attention. The critical point of halal to the product of animal origin is the animal species, the slaughtering process, the distribution until the process of preparing the product for the consumer.

This religious aspect is to help ensure food safety for consumption through adherence to good animal feeding practices at farm level and good manufacturing practices (GMP) during the procurement, handling, storage, processing and distribution of feed and animal feed ingredients in the production process. The main focus is on halal practices and safety in animal and meat production systems. Topics of concern such as animal welfare issues in livestock production, livestock processing, the concept of halal and religious issues. Halal assurance system developed by Indonesian Council of Ulama is already used in many countries around the world. It provides safety and comfort for consumers.

3.2. Sensory quality

Eating quality or palatability is determined by a single consumer response or a combination of factors such as flavor, juiceness and the tenderness of cooked meat. Assessment of sensory factor of meat is generally done by panel test by using hedonic scale. At this time some sensory indicators can be assessed quantitatively by using equipment. Indicators commonly practiced by consumers in this sensory assessment including:

1. Meat color

The color of fresh meat is one of the main criteria that consumers pay attention to at the time of purchase. Color of the meat can be determined by a meat pigment called myoglobin. Myoglobin content is influenced by genetic factors of livestock, age, feed, muscle activity, species and slaughtering techniques. Besides, the color of the meat is also determined by the reactions that occur in myoglobin. The color of fresh meat favored by consumers is a bright red color. The dark color of the meat is assessed as meat that has been stored for a long time and has been damaged. The color of the meat that has not been exposed to oxygen is a purplish red, then if it has been oxidized for several minutes it will be bright red. The bright red color may turn red or brown if there is oxidation or if the meat is stored long, or reddish-green if decay has occurred.

Ref. [16] showed no difference in semitendinosus muscle color from angus cross, bali cattle, brahman cross, peranakan ongole and simmental × PO. The results of this study are consistent with [17] that there was no difference in the color of the flesh between cattle *Bos taurus* and *Bos indicus*. Ref. [18] reported that the bright red color is the color of meat expected by consumers. The red color of bali beef is more darker (P < 0.05) than wagyu beef.

2. Tenderness

Tenderness is also a major criterion in the assessment of meat quality. If the meat is not tender, that the meat is less acceptable to consumers. Ref. [12] mention that tenderness means a quality that represents a number of structural properties of skeletal muscle proteins and is associated with all factors affecting muscle and muscle proteins (e.g. growth and development of livestock, nutrition, pre- and post- cooling, processing and cooking). The first time consumers assess the tenderness of meat is when meat first chewed. Therefore, to assess objectively based on processing that occur during mastication (the process of cutting, tearing and pressing).

Ref. [19] grouped Warner-Bratzler Shear (WBS) into four categories: very soft (WBS <3.2), soft (3.2 < WBS <3.9), intermediate (3.9 < WBS <4.6), and hard (WBS > 4.6). The strength of cut is negatively correlated with tenderness, the higher on cutting strength value mean lowest level of tenderness or tough. Ref. [20] reported that the lowest cutting strength value in male buffalo (7.17 ± 2.69 kg cm^{-2}) and female buffalo (5.89 ± 3.54 kg cm^{-2}) were present at approximately 1 year (tooth turn I0). Highest on WBS value of buffalo meat mean this meat was tough. Tenderness value of bali beef (5.8 ± 1.7 kg cm^{-2}) and brahman cross (6.3 ± 1.3 kg cm^{-2}) was not different, and angus cross beef (2.5 ± 0.3 kg cm^{-2}) had the lowest WBS value, in other words angus cross beef is more tender than other beef cattle [16].

3. Flavor

Flavor is also an important sensory aspect in consumer acceptance of meat products. It is estimated that about 1000 volatile compounds that have been identified are present in various meats (cattle, chickens, pigs, sheep and goats).

There is no qualitative difference between the types of compounds present among the livestock species, but there are differences in quantitative terms. For example, the concentrations of 3.5-dimethyl-1,2,4-trithiolane and 2,4,6-trimethylperhydro-1,3,5-dithiazine (thaidine) compounds in mutton were higher than other livestock species. While the aroma of beef is more influenced by mercapto thiophenes and mercaptofuran compounds [21]. Another indicator of this sensory rating is the amount of marbling, texture and juiceness.

3.3. Nutrient quality

Nutrients contained in the meat also entered into consideration consumers to choose meat. Meat as a protein source has a complete amino acid composition and high digestibility as well as macro and micronutrients, all of which are essential for good health throughout life. The healthiest balanced diet will include moderate amounts of lean meat, along with enough carbohydrates, fruits and vegetables, also milk and other dairy products. How much red meat should be consumed? According to the report of The Scientific Advisory Committee on Nutrition (SACN) on "Iron and Health 2010" led to new guidance on eating red and processed meat. Advice for adults, their intake is an average of 70 g daily [22].

Nutrient meats such as protein content, amino acid composition, fat content, fatty acid composition, minerals and vitamins can be chemically analyzed or biochemically. In principle a common method can be used but there are some inappropriate methods used in meat analysis. For example, to determine the protein content can be used Kjeldahl method. This method is less appropriate to use because meat protein consists of several kinds of myofibril protein, sarcoplasmic, NPN and connective tissue. For that reason BEFFE method can be derived from Germany [11]. At 100 g of beef contains 201 Kcal, 18.8 g protein, 14 g of fat, 11 mg of calcium and 2.8 mg of iron. Meat protein can help produce muscle tissue. The red color produced from beef contains a lot of iron. This iron that will produce hemoglobin which will deliver oxygen from the blood to all new muscle cells, the production of antibodies and protect the body from infection. Ref. [23] states that the average muscle protein content of longissimus dorsi aceh cattle is 15.94% with fat content of 5.63%.

The chemical composition of meat varies depending on location and function of muscle in the body. The muscles present in active organs contain more protein content compared to the muscles at the passive organs. Ref. [24] reported the content of bali beef nutrient i.e. ash content, protein content and carbohydrate levels of active muscle is higher when compared with passive muscle value (P < 0.05). While fat and water content of active muscle was low when compared with passive muscle. Ash content, protein and carbohydrate content of active muscle (0.99, 16.60, 5.99%) and the content of passive muscle respectively (0.90, 14.60, 4.32%). Fat and water content of active muscle (6.30, 70.08%) and for passive muscle (6.54, 72.99%).

3.4. Hygiene and toxicology quality

Hygiene factors in meat can be divided into two parts, namely the presence of residue in the meat and microbiological aspects. Both of these aspects are health-oriented. In consumer ratings, hygiene factors are often more important than nutritional factors.

Meat and processed products do not contain natural toxins, but can occur contamination and use of additive(s). Antibiotics can be found in meat if the animal is slaughter before the drug withdrawal (withdrawal time) runs out. Use of antibiotics is usually done in the process of treatment or use in the feed. Other residues can also occur in meat processing.

3.5. Technology quality

Consumers in addition to attention to hygiene factors are also carried out assessment of technological factors. Texture, water-binding power and pH can be felt from the hardness, juiceness and the taste of sour or tasteless. Meat experts say that technological factors are closely related to meat processing. Indicators closely related to this processing include: pH and water holding capacity.

(1) pH

The pH value of meat may indicate a deviation of the quality of the meat, since the pH value of the meat is related to the color, tenderness, taste, water holding capacity and the shelf life of the meat. The isoelectric pH points of the meat proteins are between 5.0 and 5.1 with a normal pH range of 5.5–5.8.

If pH > 5.8, then there are two possibilities of normal or DFD (dark, firm, dry). The second pH test is done at 24 hours after cutting, if pH > 6.2 means the meat is DFD, whereas if the pH is about 5.5 means the meat is normal [25]. Ref. [26] reported that meat with high pH_u has a low tenderness value.

Ref. [27] compares the physical characteristics of ongole crossbreed beef at different body weights. The results showed that body weight has a very low correlation with pH value of meat, that is, 0.192 in *Longissimus dorsi* (average pH value of 5.59) and 0.000 on *bicep femoris* (average pH value of 5.57). Ref. [18] reported that pH bali beef is no different from wagyu beef.

The pH value of meat is generally more influenced by the factor at the time of the slaughter process.

(2) Water holding capacity

Water is the most important part in meat composition. Meat contains about 75% water. Muscle protein (myofibrillar) plays an important role in water binding, which determines the quality of meat and its processed products [28].

Water holding capacity is the ability of the meat (especially myofibrillary proteins) to bind water or water added during external influences (e.g. meat cutting, heating, grinding and pressing). Ref. [29] found that water holding capacity of buffalo meat is not affected by age, but it is affected by sex during the storage period of 0, 24, and 48 hours. Result of analysis show water holding capacity of buffalo meat is not influenced by age and sex [20]. There is no difference in water holding capacity of bali beef and wagyu beef [18]. Ref. [16] also reported that there was no difference in binding power of brahman cross beef, bali cattle, ongole cross-breed cattle and simmental × ongole crossbreed cattle on *Semitendinosus* muscles.

4. Relationship of muscle microstructure and meat quality

Carcass is composed of meat, fat, adipose tissue, bone, cartilage, connective tissue and tendon. Muscle turns into flesh after cutting process because its physiological function stops. Muscle is the main component of meat constituents. All muscles have the same basic structure, consisting of muscle cells or fibers that are intertwined together in bundles and form larger groups. Collagen is the most important component related to meat texture. Collagen of old animals grow larger and they have more cross-linked connective tissues, causing the meat to become tough and less tender [12].

Muscle is composed of many bundles of muscle fibers commonly called fasciculi. Fasciculi consist of muscle fibers, whereas muscle fibers consist of many filaments called myofilaments. Connective tissue is composed of an epimysium located around the muscle, perimysium containing blood vessels, and relatively larger nerves located between fasciculi and endomysium containing amorphous component, non-fibrous tissue with fine woven binders surrounding muscle cells or muscle fibers [29].

Muscle fiber is composed of myofibrils containing many myofilaments. Myofibril is an organelle of cylindrical muscle fiber with a diameter of approximately 1–2 μm. A muscle fiber that has a diameter of 50 μm contains 1000–2000 myofibrils. Myofibril consists of segments called sarcomere. The length of sarcomere at rest is approximately 2.5 μm. Sarcomeres have two forms of myofilaments, namely thick filaments (myosin) with a diameter of 10–12 μm and thin filaments (actin) with a diameter of approximately 5–7 μm. The lighter portion of myofibril is called I band, while the thicker part is called A band. I band and A band are arranged in longitudinal parallel within muscle fibers, which causes the cross section of skeletal muscle fibers to appear transverse [12, 30]. Increasing number of muscle cells during prenatal growth can be indicated from the addition of the amount of muscle per fasciculus. Increased muscle size during postnatal growth can be indicated from the addition of muscle cross-sectional area.

Observations on histology of muscle not only result in obtaining images or descriptions of muscle tissues (existence of muscle fibers, connective tissues and intramuscular fat tissues), but also in discovering the size of the tissues (such as diameter of muscle fiber, diameter of fasciculus, and thickness of connective tissue). Nuraini et al. [20] state that the average diameter of muscle fibers of buffalo meat, which is 38.32 ± 1.9 μm, increases under 1 year of age (I_0) and reaches the highest point at the age of 3 years (I_3) with 54.95 ± 8.6 μm (P < 0.05). This is in line with the decline of buffalo meat tenderness level, which is 6.53 ± 2.89 kg cm^{-2} (under 1 year of age) to 9.63 ± 1.45 kg cm^{-2} (3 years of age). Ref. [29] mentions that many factors affect the diameter of muscle fibers, such as the level of nutrition, the rate of postnatal body weight development, the level of muscle performance and the age of livestock.

Ref. [31] describe the histology and histomorphometry of bali beef and wagyu beef. It appears that the muscle cell diameter (75.00 ± 1.72 μm) and fat cell (195.20 ± 2.17 μm) of wagyu cattle were larger than the muscle cell diameter (45.00 ± 1.89 μm) and fat cell (90.10 ± 2.69 μm) of bali cattle. Foreign tourists in Bali prefer wagyu beef than bali beef. This is partly because wagyu beef is more tender. Histologic observation results in wagyu cattle muscle illustrates that the connective tissue of wagyu beef is very little so that the meat is more tender.

Samples of muscle histology can also be used to discover the thickness of connective tissue that can be an indicator of the level of meat tenderness. Thickness of connective tissue of female buffalo at I_0 age (15.59 ± 2.00 μm) is smaller than at I_2 age (16.29 ± 5.96 μm) and at I_3 age (18.2 ± 5.81 μm) [20]. This condition illustrates that there is an increase in connective tissue as the livestock ages. It is related to the level of collagen in animal tissues. Collagen is the principal protein component of connective tissue and has a major influence on toughness of meat [30]. Collagen of old livestock is more stable against the influence of temperature change, which results in formation of thicker and larger connective tissue. An increase in livestock age is related to increased level of pyridinoline. The level of *pyridinoline* in younger livestock is lower, making collagen labile against heat.

Efforts to improve the quality of local livestock, in this case cattle and buffalo, have been conducted in various methods, both physical (e.g. aging, cold/frozen storage) and chemically (e.g. using protease enzymes). Refrigerator storage causes the split muscle fibers. Increase in period of freezer storage can result in separation of muscle fibers as well as structural damage to muscle shape caused by ice crystal formation. The fourth day of storing meat inside freezer ($-10 \pm 1°C$) shows mild damage. It is the beginning of muscle fibers cracking. On the 60th day, the structural damage of muscle fibers becomes more severe with ice crystals pressing and tearing cells. On the 75th day, the damage of muscle fibers becomes greater than the 60th day with greater intercellular distance [32].

According to [33] the diameter of muscle fibers of buffalo meat is not influenced by sex difference, but influenced by age difference during different storage periods. The data of research results conducted by Rao et al. [33]. The decrease in muscle fiber diameter occurs gradually from 0 to 48 hours of storage period inside freezer ($-15 \pm 1°C$), so as to increase the tenderness of meat during the period of aging. Freezing also affects the structure of muscle fiber diameter due to histological changes in muscle tissue during frozen storage. Muscle fibers of female buffalo that were stored inside freezer at a temperature of $-12°C$ for 35 days had less structural damage when compared to muscles stored for 79 days. Increased storage time of meat inside freezer can increase the damage of muscle fibers, so that connective tissue and the distance between muscle fibers become more easily decomposed due to the process stretching. Such damage is most likely to result in myofibril alterations.

Another treatment to improve tenderness in meat is to use enzymes, such as papain or bromelain enzymes. Related to [34], the tissue structure of beef samples not treated with bromelain enzyme is seen to have intact-shaped structures of myofibril and sarcolemma. Meanwhile, the myofibrils structure of meat samples soaked with bromelin enzyme for 1 and 4 hours looks incomplete, or in other words, has endured degradation. Descriptively, the alterations that occur in the myofibril structure indicate that giving treatment of bromelin enzyme can improve the tenderness of meat.

5. Conclusion

Summarizing the various studies of meat quality in Indonesia, it is illustrated that the quality of local meat for some criteria such as pH, water holding capacity, cooking loss, meat color, fat color, nutrient content, basically does not differ between local beef cattle and imported beef. The difference is seen in the fatty, degree of marbling and tenderness that will affect the juiceness of meat. But if it is connected with how to process the majority of Indonesian cuisine, which is wet cooking, like *rendang* and *semur*, meat quality already meet the requirements of consumer's preference. For cooking menu that uses dry cooking like barbeque it can be treated like aging with long period or using tenderizing like bromelin or papain enzyme.

Some of the circumstances causing the low quality of meat in Indonesia are most of the breeders employing cattle and buffalo, low quality of feeding, older slaughter age and handling before and at the time of slaughtering process that does not pay attention to aspects of animal welfare. The meat industry in Indonesia is only able to form two market segments namely the local market for middle to lower class consumers and special markets for hotel, restaurant, catering and franchise consumers. Efforts to improve livestock management, selection and crosses with *Bos taurus* breeds are expected to improve local livestock performance in Indonesia.

Acknowledgements

The authors thank those who participated in the various projects that led to these results, all those who provided funding support for this research and also thanks to the Open Access Publishing Fee.

Conflict of interest

The authors declare that there is no conflict of interest regarding the publication of this paper.

Author details

Henny Nuraini[1,2*], Edit Lesa Aditia[1,2] and Bram Brahmantiyo[3]

*Address all correspondence to: hennynuraini@ymail.com

1 Department of Animal Production and Technology, Faculty of Animal Science, Bogor Agricultural University, Jl. Agathis Bogor Agricultural University, Darmaga, Bogor, West Java, Indonesia

2 Halal Science Center, Bogor Agricultural University, Indonesia

3 Assessment Institute for Agricultural Technology, Ministry of Agricultural, Tidore Kepulauan City, North Malucas, Indonesia

References

[1] Kusuma SB, Ngadiyono N, Sumadi S. The estimation of population dynamic and reproduction performance of Ongole crossbred cattle in Kebumen regency, central java province. Bulletin of Animal Science. 2017;**41**(3):230-242. DOI: 10.21059/buletinpeternak. v41i3.13618

[2] Hilmia N, Noor RR, Sumantri C, Gurnadi RE, Priyanto R. Productivity and genetic diversity of local cattle in ciamis-West Java. Journal of the Indonesian Tropical Animal Agriculture. 2013;**38**(1):10-19

[3] Andreas E, Sumantri C, Nuraini H, Farajallah A, Anggraini A. Identification of GH|ALUI dan GHR|ALUI genes polymorphisms in Indonesian buffalo. Journal of the Indonesian Tropical Animal Agriculture. 2010;**35**(4):215-221

[4] Aditia EL, Priyanto R, Baihaqi M, Putra BW, Ismail M. Production performance of Bali and Ongole crossbreed cattle fed with sorghum base. Journal of Animal Production & Processing Technology. 2013;**1**(3):155-159. ISSN: 2303-2227

[5] Leo TK, Leslie DE, Loo SS, Ebrahimi M, Aghwan ZA, Panandam JM, Alimon AR, Karsani SA, Sazili AQ. An evaluation on growth performance and carcass characteristics of integration (oil palm plantation) and feedlot finished Bali cattle. Journal of Animal and Veterinary Advances. 2012;**11**(18):3427-3430

[6] Priyanto R, Fuah AM, Aditia EL, Baihaqi M, Ismail M. Improving productivity and meat quality of local beef cattle through fattening on cereals based feed with different energy levels. Indonesian Journal of Agricultural Sciences. 2015;**20**(2):108-114. DOI: 10.18343/jipi.20.2.108

[7] Setiawan D, Nuraini H. Performance of local cattle (Peranakan Ongole-PO) feed concentrate containing mulberry leave meal. Agripet. 2016;**16**(1):16-22

[8] Brahmantiyo B. Physical and chemical properties of Brahman cross, angus and Murray grey cattle meats. Media Veteriner. 2000;**7**(2):9-11

[9] Juran JM, Gryna FM Jr, Bingham RS Jr. Quality Control Handbook. New York (UK): McGraw-Hill Book Company; 1980

[10] Kaufman RG, Marsh BG. Quality characteristics of muscle as food. In: Bechtel PJ, editor. Muscle as Food. Florida: Academic Press, Inc.; 1987

[11] Honikel KO. Assessment of meat quality. In: Fiems LO, Cottyn BG, Demeyer DI, editors. Animal Biotechnology and the Quality of Meat Production. Amsterdam: Elsevier; 1991

[12] Forrest JC, Aberle ED, Hedrick HB, Judge MD, Merkel RA. Principles of Meat Science. San Francisco: W.H. Freeman and Company; 1975

[13] Halomoan F, Priyanto R, Nuraini H. Characteristic of livestock and beef carcass for traditional and specific markets. Media Petern. 2001;**24**(2):12-17

[14] Rosyidi DJ, Susilo A, Wiretno I. The effect of breeds on physical and chemical quality of meat. Jurnal Ilmu dan Teknologi Hasil Ternak. 2010;**5**(1):11-17

[15] Ismail M, Nuraini H, Priyanto R. Effect of body fatness to carcass and non carcass productivity of small frame siza beef cattle (Bali and Madura cattle). Journal of Veteriner. 2014;**15**(3):411-424

[16] Safitri A. Physical and microstructures characteristics of Longissimus dorsi and Semitendinosus muscles from local and imported cattle [thesis]. Bogor Agricultural University Graduate School; 2018

[17] Bressan MC, Rodrigues EC, Rossato LV, Ramos EM, da Gama LT. Physicochemical properties of meat from *Bos taurus* and *Bos indicus*. Revista Brasileira De Zootecnia. 2011; **40**(6):1250-1259

[18] Merthayasa JD, Suada IK, Agustina KK. Water holding capacity, pH, color, flavor and texture of Bali beef and Wagyu meat. Journal of Indonesia Medicus Veterinus. 2015;**4**(1):16-24

[19] Belew JB, Brooks JC, McKenna DR, Savell JW. Warner-Bratzler shear evaluations of 40 bovine muscles. Meat Science. 2003;**64**:507-512

[20] Nuraini H, Mahmudah, Winarto A, Sumantri C. Histomorphology and physical caracteristics of buffalo meat at different sex and age. Media Peternakan. 2013;**36**(1):6-13. ISSN 0126-0472. EISSN 2087-4634. Available from: http://medpet.journal.ipb.ac.id/. DOI: 10.5398/med-pet.2013.36.1.6

[21] Shahidi F. Flavor of Meat and Meat Products. London: Blackie Academics and Professional; 1994

[22] Geissler C, Singh M. Iron, meat and health. Nutrients. 2011;**3**(3):283-316. DOI: 10.3390/nu3030283

[23] Rotua N, Ferasyi TZ, Iskandar CD, Zuhrawati, Herrialfian, Helmi TZ. Infrared Reflectunce Spectroscopy (NIRS) prediction of protein and fat content of beef aceh cattle using Near Infrared Reflectunce Spectroscopy Applications (NIRS). Jurnal Ilmiah Mahasiswa Veteriner (Scientific Journal of Veterinary Students); 2017;**1**(4):666-673

[24] Dewi AM, Swacita IBN, Suwiti NK. The effect of muscle type and longer to the nutrition value of Bali cattle. Buletin Veteriner Udayana. 2016;**8**(2):135-144

[25] Hofmann K. Bedeutung und Messung des pH-Wertes. Fleischwirtsch. 1987;**38**(2):75-77

[26] Wulf DM, O'Connor SF, Tatum JD, Smith GC. Using objective measures of muscle color to predict beef longissimus tenderness. Journal of Animal Science. 1997;**75**:684-692

[27] Rianto E, Rahmawati MF, Purnomoadi A, Physical characteristics of Ongole bulls' meat at various body weight. In: Proceeding of Seminar on Livestock Production and Veterinary Technology. Bogor: ICARD; 3-4 August 2010. p. 301-308

[28] Price JF, Schweigert BS. The Science of Meat and Meat Products. Connecticut, Westport: Food & Nutrition Press, Inc.; 1987

[29] Lawrie RA. Meat Science. Translated by Parakkasi A. Jakarta, Indonesia: Publisher University Indonesia Press; 2003

[30] Soeparno. Meat Science and Technology. 4th ed. Yogyakarta: Gadjah Mada University Press; 2005

[31] Suwiti NK, Suastika IP, Swacita IBN, Besung INK. Histologycal and histomorphometry study of Bali cattle and Wagyu beef. Journal of Veteriner. 2015;**16**(3):432-438

[32] Kandeepan G, Biswas S, Porteen K. Influence of histological changes of refrigerator preserved buffalo meat on quality characteristics. Journal of Food Technology. 2006; 4(2):116-121

[33] Rao CA, Thulasi G, Ruban SW. Meat quality characteristics of non-descript buffalo as affected by age and sex. World Applied Sciences Journal. 2009;**6**(8):1058-1065

[34] Said MI. Isolation of bromelin enzyme from pineapple fruit and its effect on changes in beef tissue structure. Agriplus. 2012;**22**:20-25

Chapter 6

Louse Infestation of Ruminants

Borisz Egri

Additional information is available at the end of the chapter

http://dx.doi.org/10.5772/intechopen.79257

Abstract

Throughout the world, louse infestation of ruminants is an important problem that impairs the growth and performance parameters of beef, dairy and buffalo stocks. Full details of geographical and taxonomical features of blood sucking and biting louse on ruminants are discussed. The objective of the topic is to demonstrate the occurrence, biological, epidemiological and clinical importance of bovine pediculosis. At the same time, presenting factors determining the severity of infestation with blood-sucking and biting lice include the animals' age and sex and also the season. Important determination of the prevalence and rate of louse infestation among ruminants offer a survey of advances in systemic chemotherapeutic control.

Keywords: sucking and biting louse infestations of ruminants

1. Introduction

Infestations of animals with lice are medically called *pediculosis*. Origin of **pediculosis: 1885–1890; < Latin *pēdicul(us)* louse. Related forms pe·dic·u·lous [*puh-dik-yuh-luh* s]/pə'dık yə ləs/, adjective**[1].

Pediculosis in cattle occurs throughout the world, and is more common in cattle than in any other domestic animal [1, 2].

Lice infecting ruminants are wingless insects and can produce a seasonal chronic dermatitis. The most common sign is pruritus, excoriation and alopecia. The host's rubbing and grooming may not correlate with the extent of infestation. Hairballs can result from overgrooming

[1]Dictionary.com Unabridged Based on the Random House Unabridged Dictionary, © Random House, Inc. 2018

Lice species	Localization of the lice
Chewing lice	
Damalinia bovis/Bovicola bovis (cattle biting louse, red louse)	Most commonly found in the dorsum. Infestation may extend cranially to head and caudally to tailhead
Bloodsucking lice	
Linognathus vituli (long-nosed cattle louse)	Most commonly found over withers, lateral shoulders, and dewlap. May have generalized distribution over animal. In early infestations may be found in clusters
Haematopinus eurysternus (short-nosed cattle louse)	In heavy infestations, may be found over most of the body. Often found on front half of the host from ears to dewlap
Solenopotes capillatus (little blue cattle louse)	Infestations tend to be heavier in anterior portions of the body, including the ears, during warm weather. Found in distinct clusters, mainly on head and face
Haematopinus quadripertusus (cattle tail louse)	Heavy infestations may extend to dewlap or surround the eyes. Adults often confined to the tail, eggs commonly noted on tail switch

Table 1. Site predilection of cattle lice [3–5].

in cattle. In severe cases, especially in calves, the organisms can lead to anemia, weight loss, and damaged pelts. Pregnant animals may abort. Lice eggs or nits are attached to hairs near the skin. Three nymphal stages, or instars, occur between egg and adult, and the growth cycle takes about 1 month for all species. Lice cannot survive for more than a few days off the host.

Caused by several species (**Table 1**), five louse species are known to be able to infect cattle: three species of the genus Haematopinus, along with the species *Linognathus vituli* and *Solenopotes capillatus*. *Haematopinus tuberculatus* (**Figure 1**) is a typical parasite of the domesticated Asian buffalo, which is known to infest cattle as well [6] as the young animals may be

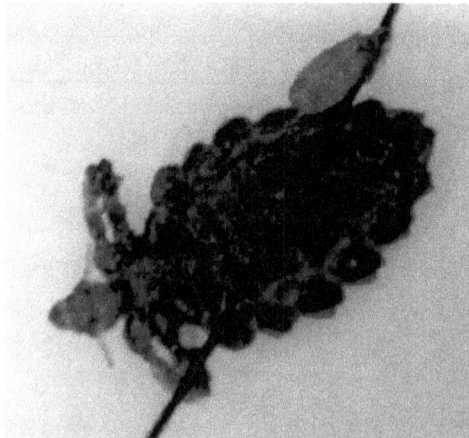

Figure 1. *Haematopinus tuberculatus* female with nit (×19.4).

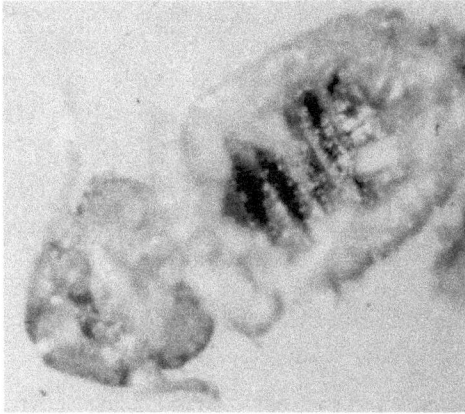

Figure 2. *Bovicola bovis* male (×26.6).

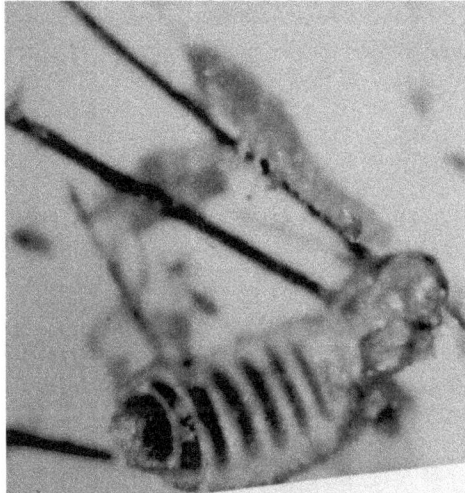

Figure 3. *Bovicola bovis* female with nymph (over) (×17.5).

infested with multiple species of lice simultaneously. *S. capillatus* and *H. eurysternus* infestations are more often recognized on mature animals, whereas *L. vituli* is more commonly seen on calves and on dairy stock. *Damalinia bovis/Bovicola bovis* is the chewing lice of the cattle [7] (**Figures 2** and **3**).

2. Life cycle

Lice undergo an incomplete metamorphosis. The life cycle takes about 4 to 5 weeks to complete. Lice lay eggs that hatch after 6–7 days. Each female deposits 20–50 (30–40) eggs (nits) during her lifetime. She deposits them one by one to single hairs. Incubation lasts 4–20 days. The eggs hatch and develop through three nymph stages to adults. Nymphs look like adults but are smaller. Adult life lasts for 2–6 weeks. Lice tend to prefer the white areas of black-and-white cattle. Off the host, most lice survive only for a few days. Survival of lice is reduced by warm weather, cattle self-grooming, loss of hair coat and good nutrition of the host [3, 4].

Lice infestations develop mostly in the colder season and peak in late winter and early spring. Skin temperature has also been correlated with the severity of louse infestation. Lice decline during the hotter season. Stabling the animals during the winter season favors overcrowding, which makes contact transmission easier. The poorer diet during winter weakens the natural defense of cattle against the lice infestations. The denser and more humid hair coat in winter offers an excellent environment for lice development as well.

In spring, food improves quickly when the herds start grazing fresh pastures. The shorter hair and the exposure to the sun reduce skin humidity, and free grazing ends overcrowding in the winter quarters, which also diminishes transmission. As a consequence, lice infestation usually recedes spontaneously during the summer season. However, a few lice usually manage to survive in some animals that will re-infest the whole herd when it comes back to the winter quarters for the next winter [3, 4].

3. Epidemiology

Lice spend their whole life on the same hosts: transmission from one host to another one is by contact. Transmission from herd to herd is usually through introduction of an infested animal, but flies or fomites may also occasionally transport lice. Up to 1–2% of the cattle in a herd can carry a high load of lice, even in the summer when high temperatures reduce the number of lice. These carrier animals are the source of reinfestation during the fall. Usually, they are a bull or a cow in poor body condition [8]. Winter housing provides the ideal conditions for the transfer of lice between cattle.

4. Clinical findings

Throughout the world, louse infestation of ruminants is an important problem that impairs the growth and performance parameters among beef, dairy stocks and buffalos. Chewing lice feed on skin and hair debris as well as on skin secretions. The other species have mouthparts adapted for piercing the skin and suck blood.

Louse infestation has been reported to cause blood loss [9], anemia, anorexia, restlessness, weight reduction of as much as 25–30 kg, diminished milk production and development of stress [6, 10–13]. The blood-sucking lice mentioned above may also be carriers of different pathogens [14]. Host animals infested with blood-sucking lice tend to keep scratching, licking and biting their skin, thus causing hair loss and skin injuries to themselves. By rubbing their body against different objects, cattle infested with lice may damage fences or trees. Such stress can reduce weight gains and milk production for up to 10% and makes the animals more susceptible for other diseases. Cattle with hair loss may be discounted at the saleyards. Skin that has been irritated by lice has a rough surface with complete loss of hair in some areas, which gives the animals an unthrifty appearance and reduces both the slaughter value and the usability of skin and hide for industrial processing [15]. In the UK, analysis of hides in abattoirs resulted in more than 80% showing some degree of lice damage. In recent years, hide or fleece damage caused by lice has been increasingly recognized as a significant effect of lice infestations. The damage is described as areas of grain loss up to 3 mm diameter that are seen on dyed crust leather [16].

For all age classes of cattle, stressors such as high stocking density, poor feed quality, gestational status, and underlying health issues are often contributing factors to susceptibility and degree of infestation.

Factors determining the severity of infestation with blood-sucking lice include the animals' age and sex and also the season. Numerous studies have been conducted to investigate correlations between the distribution of lice and the age of host animals within herds. Occurrences of bovine pediculosis do not show seasonal variation in countries with a warm climate. However, in the temperate zone and in colder regions, the most severe infestations occur in late winter and early spring, when the weather is cold and damp and the animals have the thickest coat of hair. The coat of hair serves as a habitat and shelter for lice, and provides optimum conditions for their propagation. During the year, the highest increase in the louse population occurs when cattle or buffaloes are kept indoors for the winter. In late spring, the number of lice suddenly decreases. It then remains at a low average level during the summer months when the hair coat becomes thinner, which provides a less favorable habitat for lice, because the high temperature of the skin surface and direct exposure to sunlight reduce the intensity of their development [2, 15]. Other authors have also observed seasonal occurrences of pediculosis, reporting that the population of sucking lice starts to grow in late winter, reaches its peak in the spring and its nadir in the summer and autumn months. In India, the highest 'louse index' was found in January and the lowest in June [17]. According to the results obtained by Hussain et al., the louse population reaches its highest level in February, and the environmental conditions continue to be favorable for survival and propagation of lice in March and April [9].

In a survey conducted in Pakistan [18], the prevalence of lice was significantly ($P < 0.05$) higher in cattle than in buffaloes: 144 out of 600 randomly selected cattle (24%) and only 113 out of 600 randomly selected buffaloes (18%), kept under conditions identical to those of the cattle, proved to be infected. The prevalence of louse infestation in cattle has been reported by researchers from different countries [19–21] have reported varying prevalence rates of louse infestation in cattle in association with differences in the ecological, geographic and weather conditions. Animals kept in closed management systems are not exposed to direct sunlight, which favors the survival of lice. When cattle are kept in open barns, houses with outdoor runs or in free range management system, their skin surface is directly exposed to sunlight and consequently becomes drier, which reduces the survival chances of lice and decreases the intensity of their propagation [10]. A total of 762 water buffaloes were examined. *H. tuberculatus* was found in the 11.0% (14/127) of the farms and in the 4.5% (34/762) of the animals. The presence of *H. tuberculatus* should be routinely considered because it is a cause of serious health, production and economic damages in intensive breeding buffaloes [22]. According to our observations, the female host animals and, among them, the cows showed the most severe louse infestation. Larvae of the parasite accounted for only 0.3% and adult lice represented 3.2% of all the developmental stages recovered, while 96.4% of the stages found were louse eggs. The hair samples from the bulls yielded five adult lice and 83 louse eggs, while those from the cows yielded 78 adult lice, eight larvae and 2348 louse eggs. The hair samples from the buffalo heifers yielded 12 adult lice, two larvae and 641 louse eggs, while from those of young males, seven adult lice and 16 louse eggs were recovered [18].

5. Vector significance

Lice may serve as biological or mechanical vectors for various infectious agents. *Haematopinus tuberculatus* is known to be a vector for the species *Trypanosoma evansi* and *Anaplasma marginale*. *H. tuberculatus* invasion might play a role as a vector in the intensive spreading of mycoplasma infection among buffaloes. The results of the study of Egri et al. draw attention to the importance of preventing the spread of **mycoplasma** infection and implementing control programs against parasitoses of animals [18]. The occurrence of cattle-associated Bartonella species was investigated in the cattle tail louse *Haematopinus quadripertusus* and in dairy cattle blood in the study of Gutiérrez et al. from Israel [23]. The lice were identified morphologically and molecularly using 18S rRNA sequencing. Thereafter, they were screened for Bartonella DNA by conventional and real-time PCR assays using four partial genetic loci (gltA, rpoB, ssrA, and internal transcribed spacer [ITS]). A potentially novel Bartonella variant, closely related to other ruminant bartonellae, was identified in 11 of 13 louse pools collected in summer. In the cattle blood, the prevalence of Bartonella infection was 38%, identified as *B. bovis* and *B. henselae* (24 and 12%, respectively). A third genotype, closely related to *Bartonella melophagi* and *Bartonella chomelii* (based on the ssrA gene) and to *B. bovis* (based on the ITS sequence) was identified in a single cow. The relatively high prevalence of these Bartonella species in cattle and the occurrence of phylogenetically diverse Bartonella variants in both cattle and their lice suggest the potential role of this animal system in the generation of Bartonella species diversity. To investigate louse infestation of ruminants and pathogens potentially transmitted by them, anopluran lice (n = 1182) were collected in Hungary and evaluated for the presence of anaplasma, rickettsia and hemotropic mycoplasma DNA in the study of Hornok et al. [24]. On cattle, the following species were found: *Linognathus vituli* (57%), *Haematopinus eurysternus* (38%) and *Solenopotes capillatus* (5%). *L. vituli* had a lower mean individual count/host when compared to *H. eurysternus*. On calves, only *L. vituli* was observed, with a higher louse burden than on full-grown cattle. *H. eurysternus* and *S. capillatus* were more likely to occur simultaneously with another species on the same host, than *L. vituli*.

6. Diagnosis and monitoring

Sampling involves carefully inspecting sections of skin on a representative sample of animals in the herd, either 10% or 15 animals in each group: mature cows, heifers, and calves. The best regions to inspect are head, neck, shoulders, back, hips, and tail. If sampling indicates that

B. bovis is the dominant species present, assessment of the neck and tailhead alone is sufficient to detect most infestations. If sampling indicates that *Haematopinus tuberculatus* is the dominant species present in the herds, hair samples were taken only from animals which the hair was covered with louse eggs that were easily visible with the naked eye. These hair samples were consistently collected from a 2 cm^2 area on the side of the middle part of the neck.

Although lice normally do not survive away from the host, it is possible to send live specimens by post if a suitably insulated container is used (warmed to 25°C beforehand if possible) and containing a generous quantity of suitable animal hair. Some biting lice can be maintained for at least 8 weeks and a new generation obtained *in vitro* if they are kept on filter papers in Petri dishes at 36–37°C. It is essential to maintain the humidity at 68% RH by the use of an appropriate solution of NaOH, sulfuric acid, or concentrated solution of NH_4NO_3. For short-term tests, a solution of NaCl may be used, giving approximately 75% RH as a food supply, dried yeasts with powered hair and fresh skin scrapings is supplied; it is important that these should be fresh (no more than 6 days old unless deep frozen) and from the correct host species. This maintenance technique makes it possible to test the insecticide susceptibility of strains from the field [18, 25–27].

7. Treatment

Classical concentrates for dipping and spraying with traditional contact insecticides (mainly organophosphates, synthetic pyrethroids and amidines) are quite effective lousicides for cattle. However, such insecticides do not kill lice eggs (nits) and their residual effect is usually not long enough to ensure that immature lice are killed when hatching out of the eggs. A variety of compounds effectively control lice in cattle, including synergized pyrethrins, the synthetic pyrethroids cyfluthrin, permethrin, zeta cypermethrin, and cyhalothrin (including gamma- and lambda-cyhalothrin) (beef cattle only). Many pyrethroids are lyophilic, which assists the development of pour-on formulations with good distribution [28]. Natural pyrethrins are quickly degraded, while synthetic pyrethroids such as flumethrin and deltamethrin have greater stability and a relatively long period of action [29], but they do not affect all developmental stages of the louse life cycle. Organophosphates such as phosmet, chlorpyrifos (beef and nonlactating dairy cattle only), tetrachlorvinphos, coumaphos, and diazinon (beef and nonlactating dairy cattle only) are used against lice. Certain Brahman and Brahman-cross cattle have organophosphate hypersensitivity, which should be considered when selecting a treatment compound. The compounds such as macrocyclic lactones ivermectin, eprinomectin, and doramectin are also used to control lice in cattle. Injectable macrocyclic lactones will also control biting lice, since they reach the parasites through the blood stream of the host. But control of chewing lice is usually incomplete[2]. Pour-on formulations are effective against biting and bloodsucking lice, whereas injectable formulations are primarily effective against bloodsucking lice.

---

[2]The interesting thing about it is that in the treatment of chewing or biting lice, *Werneckiella equi equi* (Denny, 1842) infestation in a foal stock in Hungary, which was treated with paste Eqvalan (MSD) (and Rintal Plus (Bayer)) at doses of 0.2 mg/kg (and 8.4 g/100 kg) body weight, respectively, after 13 days was not found with the nits of lice [30].

Multiple pour-on formulations of 5% permethrin/5% piperonyl butoxide, 5% diflubenzuron/5% permethrin, and gamma cyhalothrin are labeled for season-long control (~3–4 mo) of lice on beef and dairy cattle. Although both amitraz and spinosad are effective against lice, the last cattle products containing amitraz were removed from the USA market in 2014. Spinosad formulations for use on cattle were officially discontinued in the USA in 2010. In 2016, Bayer Animal Health introduces Clean-Up TM II Pour-On Insecticide with an insect growth regulator (IGR) pour-on for topical application to control lice on dairy and beef cattle and calves.

The compound chosen must be appropriate for the animal's age, reproductive status, and production system. The treatment of meat and dairy animals must be restricted to uses speci-fied on the product label, and all label precautions should be carefully observed. Appropriate meat and milk withdrawal times must be observed. In most countries, regulatory agencies specify tissue residue limits of insecticides and carefully regulate insecticide use on livestock. All regulations are subject to change, and pertinent current local laws and requirements should be determined before treatment [5, 27].

Research on the use of entomopathogenic fungi (*Metarhizium anisopliae*) for the biological con-trol of lice has shown promising results.

By the Parasitipedia.net for the time being, there are vaccines that will protect cattle by making them immune to lice. There are repellents natural or synthetic that will keep lice away from cattle. And there are traps for catching cattle lice. Insecticides must be used properly to achieve satisfactory control of lice. Many louse-control products require two treatments, 10 to 14 days apart. *The second treatment is essential to kill newly hatched lice that were present as eggs at the time of the first treatment and were therefore not killed.* Failure to make the second treatment in a timely manner will create problems requiring many more subsequent treatments [3].

8. Conclusions

Many factors can cause susceptibility for louse infestation (stress, pregnancy, lactation), which is important to produce optimal husbandry conditions as well as optimal animal feed-ing. Feeding cattle a high energy diet and maintaining uncrowded conditions will reduce the chances of a louse infestation. When the infested animals became asymptomatic, on the hid-den surface of the body (anal or pubic region, ridges), the louse can survive. The introducing of new animals in the herd realize necessary only after investigation of these on louse infesta-tion and use of acaricide. Secondary bacterial and viral infections may also occur, resulting in a different (e.g., mange like) lesion. The regular disinfection of infested herds and all articles that infested animals may have come in contact with are essential too, for preventing further lice infestations. Specific lice control products can be more effective than integrated pest man-agement principles, which indicate that it is preferable to use a narrow spectrum or specific product for each pest.

Author details

Borisz Egri

Address all correspondence to: egri.borisz@sze.hu

Department of Animal Science, Széchenyi István University, Mosonmagyaróvár, Hungary

References

[1] Urquhart GM, Armour J, Duncan JL, Dunn AM, Jennings FW. Veterinary Parasitology. Essex: Longman; 1987

[2] Urquhart GM, Armour J, Duncan JL, Dunn AM, Jennings FW. Veterinary Parasitology. Avon, UK: Longman Scientific and Technical, Bath Press; 1996

[3] parasitipedia.net/index.php?option=com_content&view=article&id=2398&Hemid=2665

[4] phthiraptera.Info/category/lice/animalia/arthropoda/insecta/phthiraptera

[5] https://www.msdvetmanual.com/integumentary-system/lice/lice-in-cattle

[6] Nickel WE. The economical importance of cattle lice in Australia: Advances in systemic control by pour-on method. Revue de Médecine Vétérinaire. 1971;2/3:392-404

[7] Durden LA, Musser GG. The Sucking Lice (Insecta, Anoplura) of the World: A Taxonomic Checklist with Records of Mammalian Hosts and Geographical Distributors. Vol. 218. New York: Bulletin of the American Museum of Natural History; 1994

[8] https://www.vetmed.ucdavis.edu/vmth/local_resources/pdf/misc_pdfs/ varga_article-Nov13.pdf

[9] Hussain MA, Khan MN, Iqbal Z, Sajid MS, Arshad M. Bovine pediculosis: Prevalence and chemotherapeutic control in Pakistan. Livestock Research for Rural Development. 2006;18:10-17. For author's personal use

[10] Fadok VA. Parasitic skin diseases of large animals. Veterinary Clinics of North America: Large Animal Practice. 1984;6:3-26

[11] Gibney VJ, Campbell JB, Boxler DJ, Clanton DC, Deutscher GH. Effects of various infestation levels of cattle lice (Mallophaga: *Trichodectidae and Anoplura: Haematopinidae*) on feed efficiency and weight gains of beef heifers. Journal of Economic Entomology. 1985; 78:1304-1307. DOI: 10.1093/jee/78.6.1304

[12] Loomis EC. Ectoparasites of cattle. The Veterinary Clinics of North America. 1986;2:299-321. DOI: 10.1016/s0749-0720(15)31240-8

[13] Scharff DK. An investigation of the cattle louse problem. Journal of Economic Entomology. 1962;**55**:684-688. DOI: 10.1093/jee/55.5.684

[14] Eissa SI. Some studies on Mycoplasma mastitis in cattle and buffalos in Egypt [Ph.D. thesis]. Alexandria, Egypt: Alexandria University; 1986

[15] Walker B. Cattle lice. Prime Fact. 2007;**337**:1-4

[16] Bugby A, Webster RM, Tichener RN. Light Spot and Fleck—Part 2: Animal infestation studies. Laboratory Report 186. Northampton: British Leather Confederation; 1990

[17] Rawat BS, Trivedi MC, Saxena AK, Kumar A. Incidence of phthirapteran infestation upon the buffaloes of Dehradun (India). Angewandte Parasitologie. 1992;**33**:17-22

[18] Egri B, Stipkovits L, Piszmán R. Haematopinus infestations and mycoplasma infections of water buffalo (*Bubalus bubalis*) herds in National Parks of Hungary. Journal of Buffalo Science. 2016;**5**:53-59

[19] Colwell DD, Clymer B, Booker CW, Guichon PT, Jim GK, Schunicht OC, Wildman BK. Prevalence of sucking and chewing lice on cattle entering feedlots in southern Alberta. The Canadian Veterinary Journal. 2001;**42**:281-285

[20] Nafstad O, Grřnstřl H. Eradication of lice in cattle. Acta Veterinaria Scandinavica. 2001;**42**: 81-89. DOI: 10.1186/1751-0147-42-81

[21] Topgu A. Lice (Anoplura and Mallophaga) species on cattle in the Nigde region. Veteriner Fakultesi Dergisi, Ankara Universitesi. 1999;**16**:51-55

[22] Veneziano V, Santaniello M, et al. Lice (*Haematopinus tuberculatus*) in water buffalo farms from Central Italy. Italian Journal of Animal Science. 2007;**6**(Suppl.2):926-927

[23] Gutiérrez R, Cohen L, Morick D, Mumcuoglu KY, Harrus S, Gottlieb Y. Identification of different Bartonella species in the cattle tail louse (*Haematopinus quadripertusus*) and in cattle blood. Applied and Environmental Microbiology. 2014 Sep;**80**(17):5477-5483

[24] Hornok S, Hofmann-Lehmann R, Fernández de Merac IG, et al. Survey on blood-sucking lice (Phthiraptera: Anoplura) of ruminants and pigs with molecular detection of Anaplasma and *Rickettsia* spp. Veterinary Parasitology. 2010;**174**:355-358

[25] Egri B, Nagy E. A szarvasmarha bovicolosisának kezeléséről (in Hungarian). Magyar Állatorvosok Lapja. 1995;**50**:170-171

[26] Manual of Veterinary Parasitological Laboratory Techniques. London: MAFF; 1990

[27] https://vet.entomology.cals.cornell.edu/arthropod-identification/cow-recommendations/cattle-lice

[28] Losson BJ. Chemical control of lice on cattle and other animals. Pesticide Outlook. 1990;**1**:26-29

[29] Zerba E. Insecticidal activity of pyrethroids on insects of medical importance. Parasite Today. 1988;**4**:53-57

[30] Egri B. Occurence and treatment of biting louse (*Werneckiella equi equi* Denny, 1842) infestation in a foal stock in Hungary (in Hungarian). Parasitologia Hungarica. 1990;**23**:109-113